I am 17 years old and just having a good time. Like any lucky young teenager I am indifferent to how good my life is...

Little did I to know how much things were about to change...

Cancer 'in brief'

Cancer is not a single disease. There are more than 200 types of cancer that can affect various parts of the body.

This is because cancer occurs when your body's cells begin to reproduce irregularly; and because humans are full of cells, cancer can occur almost anywhere in the body.

Cancerous cells are different to normal cells in a number of ways; but the fact that they divide and multiply uncontrollably and can travel via the blood stream infecting other parts of the body are amongst the most troublesome characteristic differences.

Another key issue is that a misbehaving cell in an organ causes different symptoms to a misbehaving cell in say your nervous system for example. Both are cancerous but the ramifications for the body will be different. Hence why there are so many different types of cancer.

If left untreated cancer will spread to other areas of the body infecting them along the way. Therefore the earlier the detection the better.

There are so many different types of cancers, and as such for diagnosis and treatment purposes they are usually grouped by the tissue area from where they originated. The four main types of cancer as at 2016 are: **Leukaemias** [blood], **Lymphomas** [immune system], **Sarcomas** [bone, muscle & body fat areas] and **Carcinomas** [the most common, occurring on external and internal surfaces like the breast and prostate].

There are said to be many causes for cancer including genetics and lifestyle but no definitive cause. People do die from the effects of cancer and people do survive using treatments [e.g. chemotherapy] that kill the cancerous cells. They say the term remission is the best you can get, you are never actually cured.

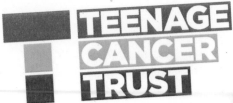

TEENAGE CANCER TRUST

CLIC Sargent

Cancer support for the young

teens:)unite
FIGHTING CANCER

dreams come true
Bringing joy to terminally and seriously ill children

WE ARE MACMILLAN.
CANCER SUPPORT

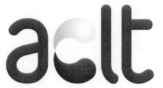

aclt

Promoting
bone marrow &
blood donation

Charities help cancer sufferers and their friends, carers and families. The emotional support and practical assistance they provide greatly assists with recovery. If you can, please support your local cancer charity they really do make a difference.

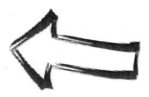

This wonderful lot helped me either during, after or ... ... both during and after. Thank you all.

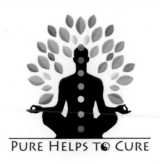

PURE HELPS TO CURE

First published in 2016 by Pure Helps To Cure &
Summer Kane Productions.

Designed Set and Edited by Studio101@d101.tv
Creative Direction by SummerKaneProductions [SKP]
Cover illustration: Jamie Williams of JW-Arts
Printed and bound by print101 London E8 1JR and
Inky Little Fingers Ltd. Gloucester GL2 8AX
Brand & Media Management Richard Kane [SKP]
Project Management Summer Kane Productions

ISBN 9780993586200 [Printed}
ISBN 9780993586248 [E-Book]

For more information or to contact the author directly visit
www.purehelpstocure.com

DISCLAIMER: The actions I take as described in this book are the choices and decisions I have made based on my experiences, reactions and research. It details the things that did and did not work for me. However each individual is different and your body can react differently to the same chemicals. I therefore urge you to investigate carefully before making any changes relating to your treatment. You can always write to me directly if you want more information or for further clarification.

(e) **charlotte@purehelpstocure.com**

All of the paper used to print this book is recycled, recyclable and or from paper manufactured from responsibly managed and sustainable sources [skp]

Contents

VITAL SUPPORT FOR YOUNG CANCER PATIENTS

Today, 10 children and young people in the UK will be told they have cancer. This news will turn their life upside down.

CLIC Sargent wants to change what it means to be diagnosed with cancer when you're young. We provide vital emotional, practical and financial support to young cancer patients and families during and after treatment, including through CLIC Sargent Social Workers and Nurses, grants and information resources.

16 to 24-year-olds who have, or have had, cancer can also share their experiences, find information and make friends at our online community: **community.clicsargent.org.uk**

Our ambition is to be there for every young cancer patient who needs us. You can help us get closer to that aim by supporting our work with a donation today.

www.clicsargent.org.uk

CLIC Sargent is a charity reliant on donations to continue our work. Registered charity number 1107328 and registered in Scotland (SC039857). 16RP189.

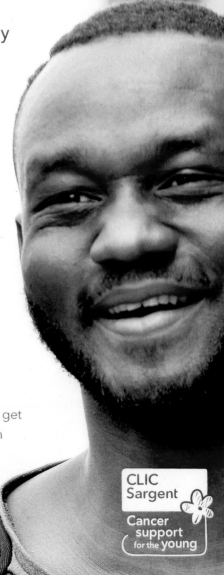

CLIC Sargent

Cancer support for the **young**

Dear Kathy

*Thank you for supporting my
project. I hope you enjoy the book.*

*Cancer is difficult and painful
and your help will help us to help
others. You are greatly appreciated.*

Best wishes

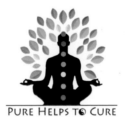

PURE HELPS TO CURE

www.purehelpstocure.com
*A Not For Profit Community Interest Company:
Registered In England & Wales | Reg No. 10099108*

a⊂lt

Promoting
bone marrow &
blood donation

www.aclt.org

Thank You

To all the **Doctors**, **Registrars**, **Nurses**
and other **wonderful** hospital staff.

I just want to take this time to say how grateful I am for everyone who helped me and worked on my case whilst I was in hospital.

As you read through my journey there will be times where frustration may shine through, they are my honest emotions that I felt at the time. It is also important for people to know how much I appreciate the Doctors, Registrars, Nurses and other hospital staff because even though I may not have agreed with how everything was handled, I am lucky enough to still be here today because of the amazing hospital team who cared for me.

I know that as a professional you have to stick to protocols and deal with things in certain ways and I commend you for this, I had to voice how I felt in order to show that there may be other ways to handle things.

Nevertheless... I just want to say THANK YOU for doing your job to the best of your ability, for helping to save my life and helping to save lives daily. To anyone who reads this book, I plead with you to support and help improve our National Health Service, it is a true world leader and a gift to our nation.

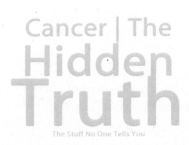

For Mum, Dad,
Tanya and Jason
thank you.

The Hidden Truth
The Stuff No One Tells You About Cancer

Hi, my name is Charlotte, I grew up in the County of Essex, South East England just outside London with my parents Albert & Jean and two elder siblings, Tanya the eldest and Jason the middle one. I saw my upbringing as a blessing, we enjoyed many family holidays and I could not have wanted for more, but of course I would not really appreciate how idyllic my upbringing had been until later in life.

This book is all about the life changing experience I went through. Not only did I contract cancer at the age of 17, but I also endured many serious side effects as a result of the treatments and medication used to combat my ailment. It was definitely an emotional time in my life.

Spoiler alert; I survive to tell the story and retrospectively everything I went through I am grateful for, as it has allowed me to view life from a totally new perspective.

My story is a prime example of how powerful the mind is; you can do almost anything that you put your mind to. I believe that anything is possible if you really want it, it may take time but if you believe in yourself and follow your instincts your outcome will be positive.

Cancer is not a pleasant experience, neither for the afflicted or their family, friends and loved ones. It is a painful journey that does not always end well. This book guides you through my experience and the measures I took to affect a positive outcome. I believe that the choices I made helped make a difference to my experience so I am sharing them here with you in the hope that you may find something in my story that will ease your journey.

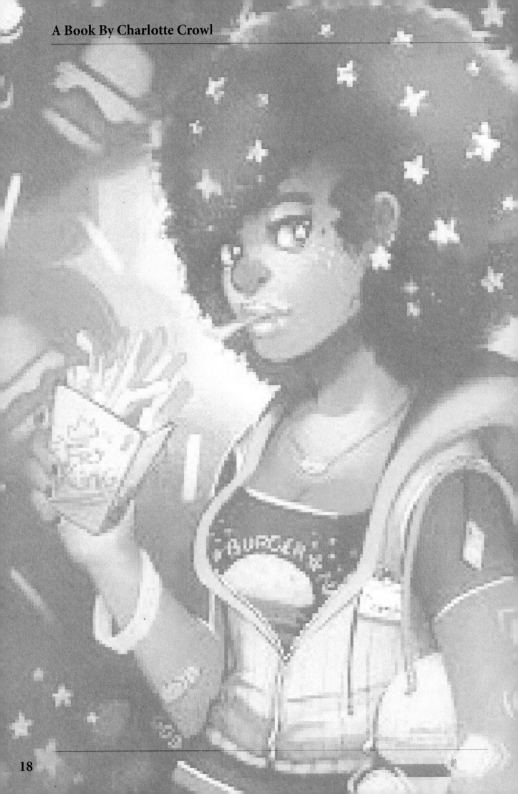

Just A Happy Girl

I once lived life without a care in the world. 'Just a happy girl' from a loving, caring and close knit family. As I advanced into my teenage years I became more independent and I felt that we as a family were not as close as we had once been... everyone pretty much did his or her own thing.

For me, I started hanging out with a different crowd of people and I would be in and around the London area a lot more. At 16 I started college, studying AS levels then on to music technology. My social diary was soon filled with extra curricular activities; night clubs, parties and bars, I'd use my cousins ID to gain entry. I started driving lessons and everything was cool... life was just fun for me.

However a consequence of my 'new busy life style' was that I had started to neglect my own health. I stopped exercising, I ate a lot of takeaways and junk food and I never drank any water. I believe that this lack of self-care was a big part of the reason I fell ill. There were other contributory factors like my unconscious mind-set; but I am glad I got to experience clubs and parties before my life changed.

2007

The Lump

For a few months previously I had been feeling a lump under my arm, and of course I mentioned this to my doctor but he said it was linked to the deodorant I had been using so I thought nothing of it. The lump eventually went away but it was to return even bigger than before. Sometimes it would hurt and give me a dead arm. I remember one night I was practically crying on the phone to my friend Drew because I was in so much pain.

One morning I felt these little nodules in my neck so I decided I would return to the doctor. He seemed quite concerned and sent me for a series of blood tests and a biopsy. At this time I did not read anything into it because besides the pain in my arm I felt like I was in good health.

I attended the hospital for my biopsy. This would be the first time I would be put to sleep, but everything seemed to run smoothly, and I was in and out of hospital the same day.

Results day came around and I was pretty oblivious as to why I needed an appointment, I thought the lump is out now so all will be fine. I remember sitting in the waiting room in my bright pink tracksuit laughing and taking pictures with my mum.

They called me into the room and that's when I 'clocked' it must be quite serious; because the consultant asked for a nurse to accompany us. We sat down and I remember the consultant saying "this is serious", I immediately thought the worst... could I be dying?

No thankfully I was not dying, although I was diagnosed with Lymphoblastic Lymphoma (cancer of the lymph nodes), which the doctor explained is curable.

My first question is "Will I lose my hair?" They say it depends on how my body reacts to the treatment. After this point all the information I am given is just a blur. I am trying to work out if this is really happening to me. The survival rate is roughly 60%, and even at this stage I see this to be very positive because it is over 50%. Mum and I then go off to a hospital side room to try and process everything, then we both cry for a little while, before leaving the hospital.

We decide it best that I speak to my college tutor as my condition will obviously affect my study. So Mum drives me to college and waits whilst I speak to my tutor. He is in disbelief but I say I will try and do some home study so I can complete the diploma. My mum then drops me off to my friend Kimmie's house where I tell her the news. I then call my cousin but it gets so emotional that I decide hereafter to avoid further tearful conversations... I will text everyone else.

Even to this day my friends still joke with me saying ' do you remember how you just text us that you had cancer', definitely one of my poor choices but no one schooled me on how I should tell people. Although I say poor choice, it worked for me at the time, so I guess really what I'm saying is whatever is best for you just do it.

Superficial (Surface) Lymphatics

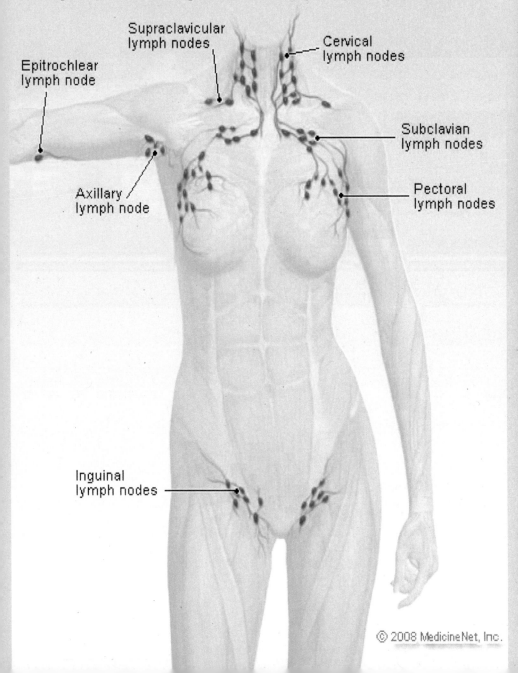

Supraclavicular lymph nodes

Cervical lymph nodes

Epitrochlear lymph node

Subclavian lymph nodes

Axillary lymph node

Pectoral lymph nodes

Inguinal lymph nodes

© 2008 MedicineNet, Inc.

"The day of my diagnosis remains so clear in my mind like it happened yesterday".

Diagnosis Day

After visiting my college tutor and texting my friends and family, I go shopping with my friend Kimmie, then off to her grandmothers. Her grandma gives me a massive bowl of red pea soup [traditional Jamaican cuisine] it tastes so good!

The last stop we make that day is to my friends aunt's house, the BBC hospital drama Holby City is on the TV and one of the characters is going through chemotherapy treatment. It's so funny that as something becomes relevant to your life you start to notice it more. I wouldn't say it's a coincidence I would just say you become more consciously aware of that particular thing.

My phone rings and it is my mum coming to pick me up. When I get in the car she tells me I am going to be admitted to hospital up in London THAT NIGHT!

I get home and pack a small suitcase, I see my dad, brother and sister and we all hug. We do not discuss the cancer I think everyone is still in shock so we just laugh and make jokes like nothing has happened.

I put my coat on, hug Tanya and Jason, and then get in the car with Mum and Dad. The drive feels like it takes forever. I am dreading having to stay in hospital, I don't really like hospitals but then again who does? Their food is nasty and they usually smell funky. We arrive outside and it is dark but the building is lit up. It is a new building and it looks amazing from the outside. Maybe this won't be as bad as I expect.

The floor I am on caters especially for young people, half the ward is for teenagers fighting cancer and the other half for teenagers with other serious illnesses.

They put me in my own private side room that looks like a hotel room in my eyes. It has a private en-suite toilet, a TV on the wall that also doubles as a monitor for the computer so I have unlimited Internet. My favourite feature in the room is the mood light *that in the future I will use for relaxation and to help me sleep.*

The ward also has a kitchen and a games room full of entertainment. Once settled I tell my parents I am ok and they can go home. I feel comfortable staying here on my own and to be honest I don't think anything has properly sunk in yet, so I just surf the internet and relax as if I am back at home.

That night they put a cannula in my hand and attach me to a drip. The cannula enables them to put medication directly into my blood stream and the drip flushes out my body and keeps me hydrated. I am also started on a light dose of steroids.

I spend the next few days taking various tests and scans so they can see what stage the cancer is at and what treatment protocol will be best for me.

Over the first week I get lots of visits from family and friends, I find this to be a great distraction as it takes my mind off all the things that are going on with my body. They say laughter is a healer and I concur; it has definitely benefited me over the years.

Within the week most of my results are back so a meeting is convened with myself, my parents, the consultant and a clinical nurse. It is a combination of good and bad news. The good news is that thankfully the cancer is not in my blood or bone marrow; however it has spread and that's the bad news. It is not just under my arm or in my neck but it is now also in my chest and stomach meaning I have what is termed as stage 3 cancer, and I will need to be on a treatment schedule for considerably longer than originally planned.

'Tis The Season To Be Jolly'

I am informed that I will be spending my Christmas 2007 in hospital, but there is a chance I can leave for New Year's Eve.

This is good because I have <u>plans</u> to go raving in London. Unfortunately I am told I will have to cancel my driving test, which is set to be in January 2008; they say I will have started my treatment by then and I will be too weak for a driving test.

On the days leading up to Christmas the ward becomes virtually empty as the hospital try to get people home for the holidays. I am not so lucky and I will spend Christmas Day 2007 in hospital. Ironically it turns out to be 'one of my favourite Xmas days ever', I love it when the family is all together, and I am about to find out that it's not about where you are but who you are with.

I wake up early on Christmas Day and get myself ready for my family to arrive. The nurse comes in to do my observations [obs] and tells me there is a present outside from Santa lol. I open it, it is full of goodies including a big MTV hoody, computer games and more. I am pleased. [*Even the little things charities do, make a BIG difference!*]

My family arrive and my mum has still cooked Christmas dinner, she even brings the rice cooker from home so she can finish off the rice and peas, pure genius! Uncle Don and my big cousin Jarrell are also here.

As a gesture of goodwill the hotel over the road prepares Christmas dinner for the ward and the guys help with the carrying and lifting. There are quite a few of us so we go and chill in the games room for a bit. I actually feel so happy this day because I am surrounded by so much love. At this point I'm thinking maybe cancer isn't too bad if it can bring everyone together like this. Then again I have yet to begin my chemotherapy so I better be careful what I wish for.

I'm feeling a bit fed up with constantly being attached to this drip so I ask if there is a way to not have it. The nurse says I will need to drink a lot more water, so from this point onwards I make sure I drink a minimum of 2 litres of water everyday. *I continue to maintain a steady daily intake of water and as a result I only need the drip for the times when they flush the chemo out of my body.*

Christmas day goes down without a hitch, I am surrounded by my family and their positive energy and laughter make for a wonderful day.

Boxing Day [26.12.07] - [30.12.07]

As the Christmas period comes to an end the ward begins to get busy again. They tell me they will need the side room for the in patients who are neutrapenic (have an extremely low white blood count). I move from my side room to a ward bed. The space is so small that I have to send most of my belongings back home. It is at this time that I am informed that I can not leave the hospital on New Years Eve as originally planned, instead I will be starting my chemotherapy treatment.

I am not happy, the thought of leaving the hospital for New Years Eve is something I have been looking forward to. To further compound my misery not only will I not be leaving but instead, I will be starting my chemo later in the afternoon. I have been dreaming of going out partying with my friends for New Years Eve, *and although it is likely that I would have been too weak to party*; the dream was real. Now there is no dream.

New Years Eve [31.12.07]

It is now late afternoon on New Year's Eve and the medical team connect the bag of chemo to my cannula, I just lie there as it runs through my veins.

They extend the visiting hours so patients and their families can see in the New Year together. I play solitaire with my dad and we make a bet that if I win three games in a row I can get a chain that I want made. I win three games in a row and start to design a chain similar to one my mum used to wear, it was my uncle's who passed when I was 5 and the chain reminds me of him.

It is approaching midnight and the nurses direct everyone around to the other side of the ward. From here we can watch the London fireworks. It is beautiful and as I sit here marvelling at the display, I am able to forget the challenges that lie ahead for me this new year. Little do I know that 2008 will either make or break me.

Chemotherapy
'the definition'

A chemical that binds to and specifically kills microbes or tumour cells. The term chemotherapy was coined in this regard by Paul Ehrlich (1854-1915).

In oncology, it is a drug therapy for cancer. Also called "chemo" for short. Most cancer chemotherapeutic drugs are given IV (into a vein) or IM (into muscle). Some agents are taken orally (by mouth).

Chemotherapy is usually a 'systemic treatment', meaning that the drugs flow through the bloodstream to nearly every part of the body.

Patients who need many rounds of IV chemotherapy may receive the drugs through a catheter (a thin flexible tube). One end of the catheter is placed in a large vein in the chest. The other end is outside the body or attached to a small device just under the skin. Anti-cancer drugs are given through the catheter.

Chemotherapy is generally given in cycles: a treatment period is followed by a recovery period, then another treatment period, and so on. Usually a patient has chemotherapy as an outpatient at the hospital, at a doctor's surgery or clinic, or at home.

However, depending on which drugs are given and the patient's general health, the patient may need to stay in the hospital for a short time.

Chemotherapy side effects depend mainly on the drugs and the doses the patient receives. Most anti-cancer drugs affect cells that divide rapidly. These include blood cells, which fight infection, help the blood to clot, or carry oxygen to all parts of the body.

When blood cells are affected by anti-cancer drugs, patients are more likely to develop infections, may bruise or bleed easily, and may have less energy. Cells that line the digestive tract also divide rapidly.

As a result of chemotherapy, patients can have side effects, such as loss of appetite, nausea and vomiting, hair loss, or mouth sores. For some patients, medicines can be prescribed to help with the side effects, especially with nausea and vomiting. These side effects tend to gradually go away during the recovery period or after treatment stops.

Hair loss, another side effect of chemotherapy, is a major concern for many patients. Some chemotherapy drugs only cause the hair to thin out, while others may result in the loss of all body hair.

Patients may feel better if they decide how to handle hair loss before starting treatment.

In some men and women, chemotherapy drugs cause changes that may result in a loss of fertility (the ability to have children). Loss of fertility can be temporary or permanent depending on the drugs used and the patient's age. For men, sperm banking before treatment may be a choice. Women's menstrual periods may stop and they may have hot flashes and vaginal dryness. Periods are more likely to return in young women.

In some cases, bone marrow transplantation and peripheral stem cell support are used to replace blood cell production when it has been destroyed by chemotherapy and or radiation therapy.

I Am Not Alone

2008

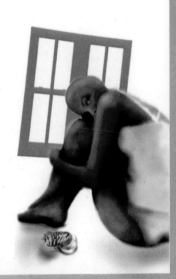

I have been in hospital now for *I think* almost three weeks. I am told that the initial rounds of chemotherapy have gone well and I will soon be discharged and sent home. This means I will be spending a lot of my time in my room in the family home so I am allowed to redecorate. One of my friends has a really nice brown and cream theme in their room so I plan my décor around the same colours. My neighbours and my dads friends are great and help with the work.

I have struck up some relationships with hospital staff members but because I have spent most of my time in a private side room I have not really interacted with any of my fellow patients. Prior to my diagnosis, I vaguely remember my sister telling me that her friend's boyfriend had recently been diagnosed with cancer. I was shocked but didn't think too deeply about it at the time. Funny how things change as it turns out he is receiving treatment here same as me.

He comes in to my hospital for day care and today is the first time I see him. His girlfriend is accompanying him and we chat. He seems full of energy as he tells me about the steroids he is taking. He shows me the marks they have caused on his stomach. He is actually the first patient I have spoken to since my admission. I feel like 'I am not alone' in my plight.

I am discharged and I return home to my newly decorated room. I am weak but extremely glad to be at home. However within days of returning I am struck down with a really bad case of diarrhoea [*I can't believe I'm telling you this but it's just the reality of the treatment I guess*]. I can not keep anything in but for me it is better than vomiting because I have a really odd phobia about vomit in general. After 3 days of this disturbing uncomfortable experience I have no choice but to return to the day care unit. They do not have any space on the cancer ward so they give me a side room on the other side of the ward. I have lost a lot of weight, I look in the mirror and see a stranger staring back at me. I hate mirrors right now.

It is during this period that I have one of the most terrifying experiences of my life...

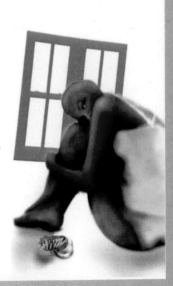

Meet Cherona

The diarrhoea episode continues to plague me. My steroid dose is increased and boy do I know it. I am totally obsessed with food. Immediately I wake up I begin planning what I will be eating for every meal. Every morning I wake up at 4am and get my mum to make me half a pack of noodles whether we are at home or in the hospital. This is currently my routine; sleep, medication, toilet and food. If I'm not sleeping then I'm eating, if I'm not eating then I thinking about food. I'm obsessed. It must be the steroids.

It is during this period that I have one of the most terrifying experiences of my life… Her name is CHERONA and she is paranoid, evil and doesn't listen. 2% of the time she is happy but 98% of the time she is anything but happy. She turns up when she feels like it and the worst part is that she controls my mind and drives me crazy. In the morning when the doctors come around, I have a list of stuff I wish to tell them, but my mind always goes blank when they arrive.

Tonight everything is getting too much and Cherona takes full control. She rings my cousin Corrine and tells her "bye, it's my time to go". My mum and dad call the nurse as I utter the words "I don't want to live no more can you just give me a drug to make it go away". It feels like I am present but someone else is talking through my body. The nurse handles the situation really well and calms me down.

My mum tells me that if I wanted to not be here I wouldn't, she is right but she does not understand that I am currently possessed by Cherona. Aunt Lizzie is here to see me, we pray together, I feel a lot better.

It is a weekend and this means I will not be seeing a registrar until the Monday. Cherona has gone for a while so I take this opportunity to write down my questions for the doctors, I also convey the list to my mum so that if Cherona should up and present herself Mum can still convey my points to the registrar.

It is now the early hours of the morning and Cherona is up and awake, but this time she is really happy although slightly deluded, this is still a welcome change, although I'd much rather she was asleep. Cherona wakes up my mum and tells her she has to shower NOW because she will feel too weak in the morning. She sings in the shower and thinks her voice is great, maybe even x-factor material. My mum suggests I wait and see how I sound in the morning.

Morning comes around and I feel like myself again, I apologise to mum for keeping her up so I could shower. I ask her can I sing? She replies "No" and we both start to laugh.

The registrars are approaching and I am able to relay my list to them. I explain how the steroids have messed with my emotions and I ask if I can be taken off them. The answer is... No *because steroids play a very important role in my treatment, they actually shrink the cancer cells.*

There is however some good news, I am to be discharged and can return home as there is 'no trace' of an infection in my blood system, *infections are an unwanted chemotherapy treatment side-effect, your chances of contracting an infection increase greatly during your treatment program.* However before I can leave I must visit with a psychologist for an assessment. Cherona had earlier told the nurse that I didn't want to live anymore. So my mental state has to be evaluated to ensure I am not a danger to myself.

Great, maybe this can at least help me to get my steroid dose reduced. I begin to collect my things together ready for my discharge and wait for the psychologist. *It turns out I need not have bothered.*

Here he comes, he looks quite young maybe he is still a student. *I'm no trained psychologist but I do have common sense and sensitivity when it comes to dealing with delicate matters. This man lacks both.*

He sits in front of me with his notepad and pen and the first question he asks is "Why do you want to die?". I'm shocked by the bluntness I can't answer I just give him a look as if to say 'really, did you just ask that'. He packs up his things and leaves, just like that. My mum and I are in disbelief that he has just asked that. Anyway I am glad to be getting back home to my newly decorated room so I won't let him ruin my day.

I am now back at home and my sister Tanya is down for the day, I don't know why... but I feel as if something evil is trying to get me. We get fish and chips from "oh my cod" their food is the best but today my mind is not right, I barely finish my food. I go to the bathroom and 'lo and behold' Cherona is back with a bag full of weird ideas. "People can die from swallowing tissue so get eating" I start eating tissue. I then eat a piece of the money plant that is in the bathroom. The bathroom light switch is on a long string and I try to wrap it around my neck, this is not working!

I go back to my bedroom and I shout out "Mum, bring me up a cup of hot chocolate"

Right now my eyes are closed and I feel tingly all over, it feels like this is it, my time has come, my body is giving up on me. I am not scared to die, I actually feel ready and at peace.

I'm not quite sure what is happening. It is like I am having an out of body experience. I envision my self lying on the bed but it is as if I am standing next to the bed looking over my body. I then envision my uncle who passed away when I was five, he tells me it is not my time. I hear footsteps coming up the stairs, it is my mum with my hot chocolate. I regain consciousness and just lie here trying to work out what has just happened. If I tell anyone what has just occurred I may get sectioned, but I do tell my mum pleading with her not to tell the doctors.

Shall I go to the hospital? Has this tissue swallowing exercise damaged me? No I will be fine, time for sleep.

I must have slept through the night because it is morning now. I have to go to the day care center today to get my pic line inserted. *A pic line goes through the inside of your arm and sits at the top of the heart. It makes it a lot easier to take blood from the human body and when used in reverse gets the drugs into my blood stream a lot quicker.*

This piece of apparatus is great for me. It means no more cannulas for the duration of my treatment. My hand is practically blue from where my skin has been bruised from all the cannulas I have had since my first hospital admission, so it is a welcome change.

Now it's time for some scans and further tests. [They will phone me when the results are in]. All done now and I'm good to go home.

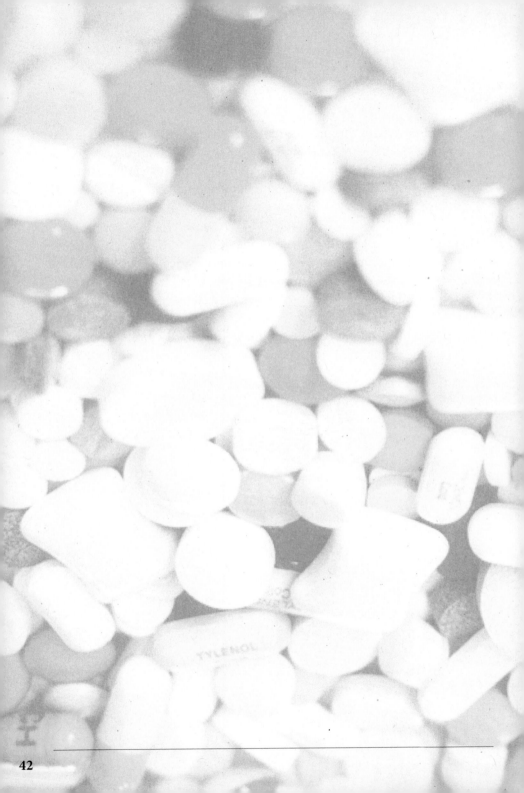

No Bed Of Roses

I have been home from hospital for about a week. Today I am in my bedroom relaxing with Mum, Tanya my sister and my cousin Corrine. I have recently become obsessed with keeping my hands clean. *I may have acquired this new found habit as a consequence of my recent hospital stay; after adopting the strict hand washing regime all hospitals understandably employ.*

I must wash my hands. I go to the bathroom and do just that. I return to my room not quite with it. My mind is in some sort of a trance. Nothing is registering, everyones voice seems to be repeating like a CD when it sticks.

The phone rings and this snaps me out of the trance. It is the hospital, I need to come in as something is showing on my scan. *Oh no here we go again!* We leave home and drive to the hospital. On arrival I am given another scan. The scan confirms I have a lung infection. I'm gutted, I don't feel any different to normal really but I am admitted to a side room.

We all go up to the ward and sit in the games room where my other friend Tia is already waiting. I must use a wheelchair as I am quite weak. Not sure who is pushing but it is welcomed. The accumulative effect of the past few months is taking its toll and I have lost a lot of weight.

This cancer thing is no bed of roses, it's more like lying naked on a bed of thorns.

The lung infection escalates quite quickly and at times I have to use an oxygen mask to help me breathe. I feel pain all over my body. I inform the medical team and I am visited by a pain doctor. I am given liquid morphine plus two morphine tablets that are purple and orange. The two forms of morphine are added to my ever burgeoning medication chart.

The morphine has a calming effect on my body. I am however, losing all sense of time. Days are merging into each other. Today I am hallucinating weird stuff. I keep seeing a giant Pudsey bear moving up and down the wall and it looks like he is raining transparent jelly spiders at the window. I'm not scared just some what confused.

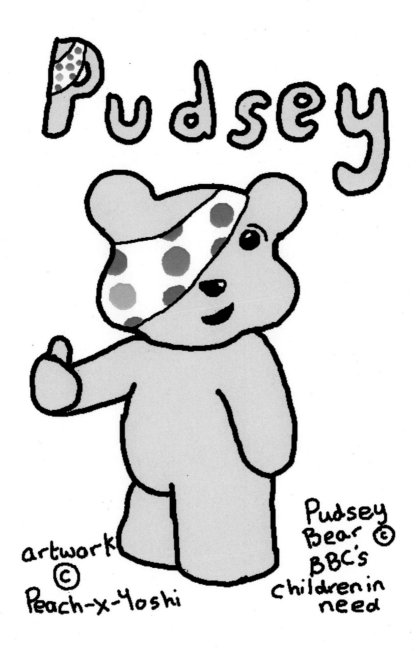

artwork
©
Peach-x-Yoshi

Pudsey
Bear ©
BBC's
children in
need

Medication Reminder Chart: Charlotte Crowl

Medicine name & strength		Medication times and how much to take				Reason for prescribed medication	Special instructions
		Morning	Lunch	Evening	Night		
Co-trimoxazole (Septrin)	480mg tablets	One		One		To prevent pneumonia	Only on Mondays and Tuesdays
Omeprazole	20mg capsule	One				Reduce stomach acid	
Dexamethasone	2mg tablets	Two	Two	Two		Part of Treatment	Take this dose up to and including the 21-01-08
	500mcg tablets	Three	Three	Three			
	2mg tablets	Two	Two			Part of Treatment	Take this dose on the 22 - 24.01.0
	500mcg tablets	Three	Three				
	2mg tablets	Two	Two			Part of Treatment	Take this dose on the 25 – 27.01.
	500mcg tablets	Three					
	2mg tablets	One				Part of Treatment	Take this dose on the 28 – 30.01 27 -28 then stop
	500mcg tablets	One					
peridone	10mg tablets	One	One	One	One	Anti-sickness	Take only if needed
nsetron	8mg tablets	One	One	One	One	Anti-sickness	Take only if needed
histerone	5mg tablets	One	One	One		Prevent periods	
ose	Liquid	10ml			10ml	To treat constipation	Take regularly when needed

Allergies: Nil known Drug Allergies

Short Back & Sides

It is time for me to add another chemotherapy drug to my treatment schedule. This one is called "Daunorubicin", it is red in colour and one of its side effects is hair loss, *my greatest fear*. I will therefore need a wig. The wig lady comes around and I choose one free wig, I go for a short bob.

I am scared that I will wake up one morning to find all my hair on the pillow. Cherona is also back and she is insisting that my mum cut all my hair off. Mum doesn't want to comply saying "it is just the steroids talking you will regret it in the morning". Cherona is persistent she will not let it go. Mum cuts my hair into a bob and I go to sleep.

I get up in the morning and go to the toilet. I wash my hands and look in the mirror. Who is this person staring back at me? Where is my hair? I question my mum and she informs me of the conversation we had the night before. To be honest I am just glad she has not shaved it all off.

Over the next few days I notice that I lose more hair than usual when brushing. The effects of the drug have kicked in and my hair is thinning. It doesn't look very good and I am upset. I think it is best I shave it all off.

One of the games room co-ordinators has sheers here, *I guess it is quite a common thing on a cancer ward for patients to want to chop their hair.* She shaves it all off and I keep a lock of hair for myself. I go to the bathroom so I can check out my new look. I burst into tears, who is this person in the mirror? I have lost so much weight and I feel so 'un-pretty'. The confident girl who once existed is now lost.

For the first time I can see how unwell I have become. I pick myself back up and try and look at the positive side, I tell myself 'there is always sunshine even if it is hidden by clouds'.

I look back in the mirror with my new found positive attitude. I have a perfect head shape but I still don't let anyone but my immediate family see me bald. I build up a pretty impressive wig and hat collection whilst in hospital, but to be honest as soon as I am alone I can't wait to take the wig off and let my head be free.

Today my cousin Corrine and friend Chris are visiting me. I decide to pull off my wig right there and then without pre-warning. I do it and start laughing. Corrine laughs too, Chris just looks. I think he is a little shocked or maybe it is a stark reminder of what I am going through.

I don't say anything to them, I am actually feeling good as I always do when I take off my wigs. This is a milestone moment for me. I am coming to terms with my baldness. From herein I feel comfortable without a wig and everyone on the ward is in the same boat, so this makes it even easier for me to 'go natural'. I receive lots of compliments saying how the shaved look suits me; and these are welcome, although I still miss my hair.

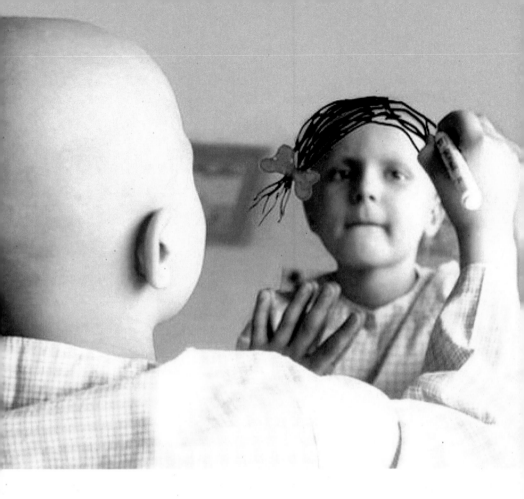

dreams come true
Bringing joy to terminally and seriously ill children

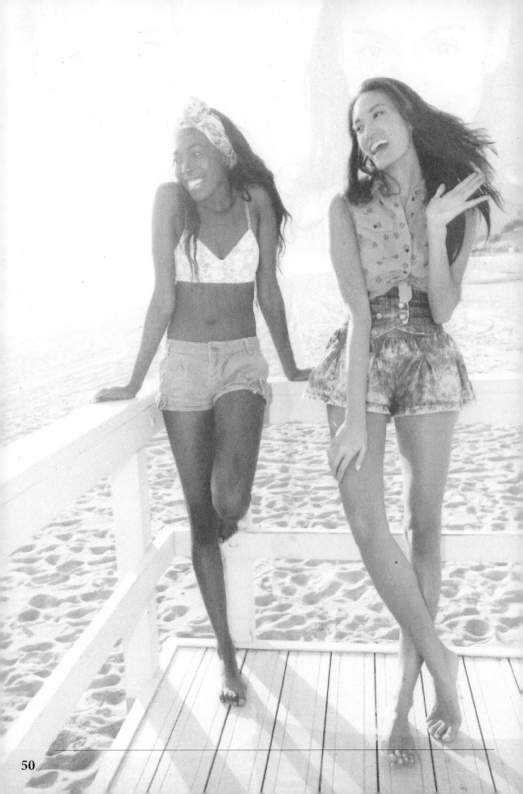

First Encounters

Today I am told that my steroid dose is to be reduced. Over the next few days I begin to regain a sense of self. It is now that I realise how much of a blur the past few weeks have been. The reduced steroid dosage is having the desired effect and I am feeling more like myself.

I am moved from my side room to a ward. The antibiotics have also had the desired effect and my lung infection has gone. I am given platelets over night. I wake up with some serious energy, I feel so good everything seems a lot better.

There is a girl in the bed opposite me called Savannah, we talk, she is the same age as I am. We hit it off. This is the first time I encounter Savannah and it is so nice to have someone to talk to who is similarly afflicted.

She will became one of my closest friends whilst I am ill, when either of us are in side rooms one will visit the other and we talk for hours. We often get into trouble with the nurses as you are not meant to leave your room whilst your immune system is as low as ours.

Having Savannah transforms my hospital experience. Days are no longer so long. Having her is like being on the beach with your best friend; although we are not on the beach we are in a dull hospital with cold hard surfaces and cold walls, but it feels a lot better when we are together.

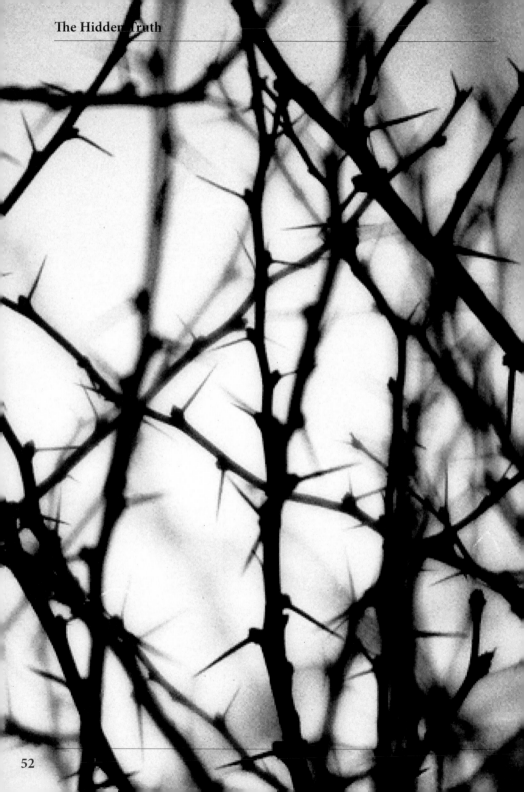

Bed Of Thorns

New day and hooray [not], it is time for my next batch of chemotherapy. This comes in the form of a drug called Methotrexate. It is categorised as one of the strongest drugs on the chemo treatment schedule and the list of possible side effects reflect this.

I have had Methotrexate before. They use it when performing a lumber puncture, they inject it in to you to protect the fluid that surrounds the spinal cord and brain. The difference this time is that the dose is much larger. They run it through my veins over a 24hr period.

It is then flushed out of my system. They tell me this will take anywhere between 3 and 10 days. I don't fancy staying on this ward for ten days attached to this drip. So I drink plenty of water in order to assist getting the drug flushed out of the body quicker.

After only one day of flushing, the registrars are amazed that my bloods are showing as fine, it means I will be able to go home. Just to be sure they double-check my bloods, yes they are fine. I feel a sense of pride that my body has flushed out the drug so quickly; that decision to drink water daily and regularly is paying dividend. I am so pleased to be going home.

I've been home for a few days now. Today my mouth and throat are covered in ulcers [a known chemotherapy side effect], and this is making it extremely hard to eat or drink anything. My mum has to blitz all of my food for me because chewing is way too painful. A few more days pass and I regain some strength and energy and feel pretty good.

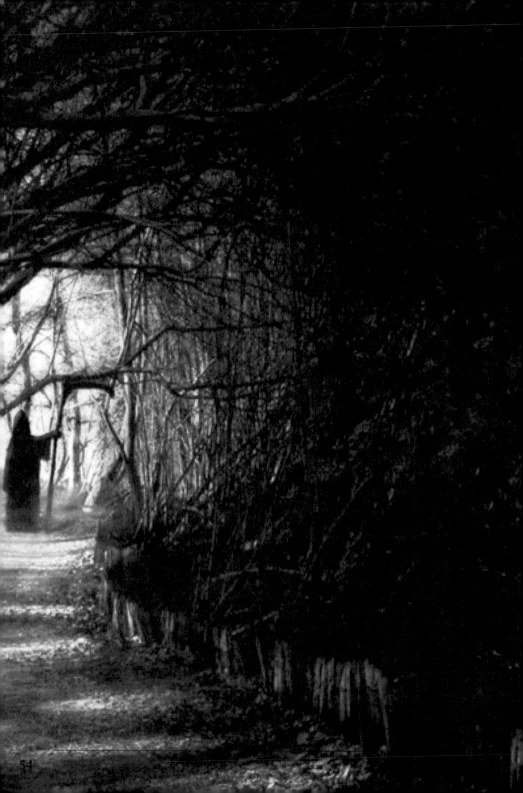

The Long Dark Tunnel

It is now late March 2008, less than a month until my 18th birthday. My health situation is 'not great' to put it mildly but I am determined to celebrate and make it memorable.

My cousin and friends are planning something for me, I'm not exactly sure what it is yet but I know I'm going to have to wear something, so I go shopping with my mum to get a birthday outfit.

The next morning I try on the outfit and take a nap. I wake up... oh no what is this? I can't feel one of my arms it is dead. I try to lift it with the other arm but once I let go it just drops. I call my mum, she holds up my arm and when she lets go it just drops again.

We both start to laugh, then we stop as we realise that this may be serious. I get up to go to the toilet and my walking is all amiss. I stagger and my speech is slurred, you'd think I was drunk.

Mum says we need to go to the hospital quickly, no time for an ambulance she will drive. She calls the hospital and gets me downstairs and into the car. She goes next door to get my neighbour to come with us to the local hospital. We arrive and I get in a wheelchair. My neighbour takes the car back home because this is clearly going to be an overnight stay at best.

I reach the ward and by now my speech and mobility have decreased to about 40%. Mentally I am still in situ *although to this day it is a mystery to me how I managed to remain so calm.* I am put in a side room and await the consultant.

My body is now pretty much fully shut down, I have 'no' body control, I can not speak and it is hard to swallow my saliva let alone anything else. As I lie here I can hear the nurse and consultant speaking, they think I am psychologically challenged at present. They discuss my case and I can hear them saying either the cancer has spread to my brain or it is a side effect as a result of one of the chemotherapy drugs.

I am not medically trained but I know or is it feel? Either way I am sure it is not the cancer that has spread to my head causing my body to shut down in such a short period of time.

What I do know is that even though my last batch of chemo was nearly 2 weeks ago, it was extremely strong and seemed to flush out of my system "alarmingly" quickly.

Great! I have just self-diagnosed myself and ascertained that it is not the cancer but the chemo, but I can not even share my thoughts with anyone as I can not string two words together. I make a conscious decision there and then that where my health is concerned I will no longer be putting all my faith in 'the system'.

They tell me I must have a MRI scan, and I think not again. I really dislike these. They put you through that noisy claustrophobic tunnel whilst your head is caged down and you have no control over your body. For me it is an absolutely horrific experience.

I make sure I let them know I am not happy about the idea of a scan. I am quite distressed, so much so that I am sedated and my mum is allowed to accompany me into the MRI room alongside the medical technicians performing the scan.

After the MRI scan the hospital staff contact the London hospital where I have been receiving my chemotherapy treatment and arrange for me to be transferred back to them.

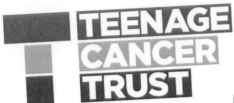

TEENAGE CANCER TRUST

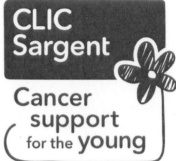

CLIC Sargent

Cancer support for the young

teens:)unite
FIGHTING CANCER

dreams come true
Bringing joy to terminally and seriously ill children

WE ARE MACMILLAN.
CANCER SUPPORT

aclt
Promoting bone marrow & blood donation

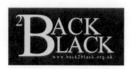

²BACK BLACK
www.back2black.org.uk

The Fight Back

I remember when I was younger I always wanted to go into an ambulance with the blue flashing lights on. This however is not how I imagined it to be. I am laid flat down with lots of wires coming off me plus some suction thing for my mouth because I can not swallow unaided.

We arrive at the hospital in no time. The ward is not prepared, I think they have underestimated the severity of what is happening to me. I am not even given a side room instead I am taking up two bed spaces on an open ward. The curtains are pulled across and there are lots of staff around. My Dad arrives and confronted with this scene is unable to hide his concern, it is clearly visible on his face.

I just smile at him. I know it is my job to keep strong for my family and myself. If I remain calm and show no fear it will reduce the stress for them.

The doctors are confused they have not seen this type of side effect from this chemo drug before. One of the consultants seems pretty sure that I will be up and back to normal within 3 months. *Now what he said was far from the reality of what really happened. Yet I believe to this very day that those words boosted my positive mentality and set me on my road to recovery. This is because he was the only person who seemed sure of themselves and it was the first positive feedback I had pertaining to this situation. I think it also gave my parents faith that everything would be ok.*

I can not pronounce a word let alone string a sentence together. It's been this way for about six hours. I know that my will power will pull me through. I struggle and manage to tell my parents "I love you".

I am finally moved into a side room where they attach a catheter and food tube to me. I go to sleep. This next morning a neurology professor comes to see me. He carries out some reflex tests and leaves the room looking puzzled. Later I speak to the consultant who has come to explain the neurologists findings, he tells me that my case confuses them because parts of the body that normally do not respond in this type of situation are responding.

My brother who is away on holiday calls my mum to see how I am doing because he has seen me in his dream; it is like we have some sort of telepathic communication going on.

My mum knows I do not want any visitors unless it is immediate family, I'm just not up to it. I don't know how I look but judging by all the wires I am hooked up to, it is not a good look.

I am heavily sedated and this lasts for a few days, I don't really remember how many I just sleep most of the time. My mum tells them to reduce my sedatives, she knows there can be little improvement whilst I am sedated.

My sedation begins to wear off and even though I can not speak my personality is still able to shine through. The outpatient staff come and visit me. They always know how to put a smile on my face, especially Connie.

Mum tells me Savannah is in and on the ward. Mum wheels Savannah round to see me. I can't speak so I just smile. She looks at me and starts crying whilst asking me how I can still be smiling? I want to tell her to not cry and give her a hug, but of course I can not move or speak. My mum hugs her and tells her everything is going to be ok.

I start my physiotherapy program; well I say start, I can't really do anything, they come in and move my body. I think this will help train the muscle, nerve and brain signals. There is a handsome trainee physiotherapist attending my sessions. It is definitely morning motivation... I have a permanent smile on my face.

I am moving to the biggest room on the ward as it is now free. My mum leans over me to get something and my nose stud gets caught on her top and pulls out. All I can do is make sounds to signal what has happened, it is really frustrating. It takes a good 20 mins for Mum and Dad to realise. Dad asks me a series of questions telling me to blink once for yes and twice for no. I can not however control my blinking effectively. *We always look back now and laugh at that moment; it also acts as another reminder as to how far I have come.*

I feel really hot all the time and need a fan on 24/7. I barely wear many clothes because with all the wires attached to me it is difficult to put stuff on. I wear just a vest top, girl boxers and socks, which all have to colour co-ordinate. My daily outfit is one of the few things I have control over. It is currently an obsession to make sure I am colour co-ordinated.

I do not like the fact that I can not even push myself up on the bed or roll over. I know how to, I can even visualise myself doing it, but the signals are not operating my body.

My mum has to help me with absolutely everything; I am like a new-born baby. I am beyond grateful for her constant assistance. Not once does she complain or show a grudge, my mum is definitely the greatest woman I know. *Before any of this happened to me I was a very proud and private person. This experience has taken away all my self-assurance but I have gained a lot of gratitude.*

Most of the time when you have or can do something you take it for granted forgetting not everyone has the same luxury. Well as I lie here hopelessly in this bed I realise in life that I have always wanted more. I have never taken the time to truly appreciate the things I have.

Instead of thinking why me and feeling sorry for myself I need to look for the positives. This mind-set in this moment in time is what I need to continue pushing for better. The fight back has began. I have been slowly building to this point for some time now and today it seems to have clicked.

The amount of love and support I receive from my family and friends, is astounding. It draws me closer to people who I was not as close to prior to being ill. More importantly this support helps to give me the strength to fight back.

My first aim is to get myself off the food tube! At present I am not even able to choose what I want to eat; I can not drink, as I am 'Nil By Mouth'... it is written on my chart and above my bed. It has been weeks since I have tasted anything in my mouth. It is a weird feeling always feeling full when you have not even eaten. I think they give me too much food because my belly is always bubbling and I feel over full. Plus the food tube is taped down on my skin and can pull and hurt.

Today is Sunday and the nurse wants to change my bed but I am too weak to move. She brings the hoist to help her move me. What a traumatic experience! Usually when I am weak the nurses just help me off the bed, but this nurse thinks the hoist is a better option, as it is "safer".

She straps me in and begins to hoist me up into the air, it is so uncomfortable. I get my aunt Lizzie to follow my movements with the fan; if the fan goes off me, I panic because it feels like I am burning up. The nurse does not even know how to operate this contraption properly and leaves me suspended in the air as she works it out.

Phew all done now. There is no way I am getting back in that contraption, not for anything or anyone.

I start my speech therapy, this is my first session and I am allowed to have yogurt. I'm not a big fan of yogurt but it feels like the most amazing feeling; to be able to taste something in my mouth again. I am also allowed to try some soup. My sister Tanya works in Marble Arch and she brings me some red pea soup from Mr Jerks on Wardour Street, London. Oh this is so tasty!

The physiotherapy and occupational therapy are a lot more intense. I can now stand up. This confirms to me that my mobility can be fully restored. It is going to take a lot of time and effort but as long as I keep consistent and persistent I will see constant results. My walking is currently similar to a new born learning to walk; it isn't until they are 3 or 4 that it becomes fully smooth.

There is however a big difference between a new born and an almost fully grown adult like myself, to a newborn it comes naturally and once their patterns have been formed it is automatic. When you are older you don't actually learn to walk the same way because those patterns have already been created so you learn a different way.

To further complicate things I already know how to do all of this in my head but all of the pathways from my brain to my muscles have been wiped. There is a risk that bad habits will creep in because it is not a natural learning process and some parts of my body are weaker than others causing me to compensate by using the stronger parts.

Plus there is the fact that I am still fighting cancer using some very strong drugs that zap my energy. There's the mental aspect too, i.e. the fear of how others will perceive me.

I want to be home for my 18th birthday and ideally not stuck in a hospital bed. The next aim is to be able to walk unaided and to climb some steps. This way I will feel safe and comfortable to get around.

Three days before my birthday and they are telling me that they do not think I am ready to go home on day release. I am upset but at the same time relieved. Mentally I am not yet ready to face going home. I am used to my current surroundings, I am comfortable in the hospital room, Going home will require a lot of readjustment.

The ward staff get to hear that I will not be going home for my birthday. "Don't worry, we will make it nice for you"

One day to go until my 18th birthday and my cousin and friend come in to see me, they have presents from themselves and my other friends. They also have a big card, which has some really nice messages written inside, plus a cake with a picture of me in my pink tracksuit on it. I can not say much but I appreciate the company as I listen to all the stories of what everyone has been up to. It is a nice time and my mum is able to get a little break and some time to herself.

Mum is able to get a little break and some time to herself.

19.04.2008

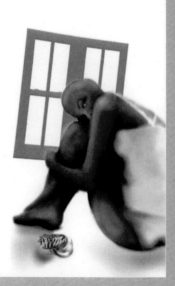

My 18th Birthday

As a kid you can't wait to grow up and turn 18. I am finally legal to drink and club and luckily I experienced all that before falling ill. I feel humble today and for the first time I am actually truly truly grateful for seeing it through another year.

The games room leader has decorated my room with lots of birthday stuff. It is time for my reiki and reflexology session, this is so lovely and relaxing. Surprisingly I get lots of visitors through the day, my room is continuously full. It is one of my most memorable birthdays. It is unplanned yet I feel an unlimited level of love and support.

My Dad brings me a gigantic elephant teddy. All the guys from my parents workplace have contributed. There is a staff shirt with a message from each staff member written on it. What a lovely gift.

Next in is my brother *accompanied by Cherona*. My brother has just returned from a snowboarding trip and he has a new piercing. I get upset with him and become really persistent that he removes it. I ban him from the hospital until he takes it out. I say I, it is actually Cherona with the lofty ideas.

Most people would feel pushed away and probably avoid seeing or talking to someone who treats them in the way I have just treated my brother. My family have to put up with a lot as I have constant mood swings. As always they are very supportive and understanding. They only show me love and do not let any other emotion shine through.

I care way too much about what other people think of me!

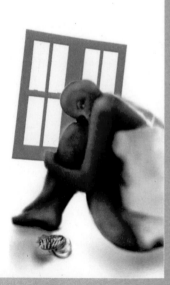

The Wheelchair

Great Aunt Maria is over from Jamaica and has come to visit me accompanied by her son Max who lives here in the UK and is a black cab driver in London. *Earlier this morning I made sure I looked as good as possible because I knew they were coming and Aunt Annie will soon be returning to Jamaica where my grandparents will be expecting a full report of my progress; so I want to look my best so as not to add to their concern.*

Max has some great news, he is getting married later this year. I tell him I will be walking unaided by then.

Up until now I have avoided getting in the wheelchair unless I am too weak or sedated. Everyone tells me how good it will be for me to get fresh air, but that will involve me using the wheelchair and my pride thus far has been a major obstacle. Previously when I had to use the chair I didn't mind because it was down to me lacking energy, but now it is down to my mobility. I don't want people staring at me casting judgements like; what happened to her? Why is she in a wheelchair? I wonder if she can walk?

I care way too much about what other people think of me! Today I need to go get new trainers to do my walking in. My dad has only gone and polished my trainers lol, he means well, but they no longer look like trainers but more like school shoes. *This is definitely one of those funny stories, which we still talk about now.*

My parents and I go to the West End, which is literally down the road from the hospital. It is actually interesting to see which shops actually cater for wheelchair users. As I am wheeled down from Tottenham Court Road to Marble Arch no one really pays attention to me, it feels great for peoples attention to be elsewhere for once.

The other side of it though is that people have total tunnel vision and no awareness of what or who is around them. They suddenly just stop in the middle of the pavement, I joke and say we need traffic light signals on the pavement so we can get some order in place. If people stare at me I stare back and put my legs out straight so they can see my legs are still operational.

I am even more self-conscious because I have put on weight from where I have been on a food tube and don't really move around. The steroids are also defiantly having an impact on my appetite and I now love food to the maximum as I am off the food tube and free to eat by mouth normally. I am only wearing jogging bottoms because my other clothes are uncomfortable and don't fit.

The steroids have also made my big eyes appear huge. I keep doing this annoying thing that I can't control; i.e. when I meet new people or explain something I open my eyes wider, it is like I have a constant surprised look on my face. *Sometimes I think I still do it now, when I'm concentrating really hard.*

I am now overcoming my foolish pride and I am a more regular wheelchair user. I love going out to get fresh air. I leave the hospital a little more often for wheeled trips around the Capital. There is less than a small chance I will bump into anyone I know, plus even if I do they probably will not even recognise me. It is one of my greatest fears, people from my past seeing me in this state. It is a motivating force; I must get myself back on point as soon as possible.

I don't want people staring at me casting judgements like; what happened to her?

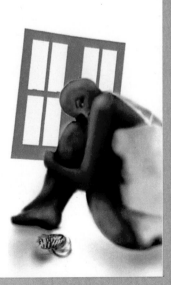

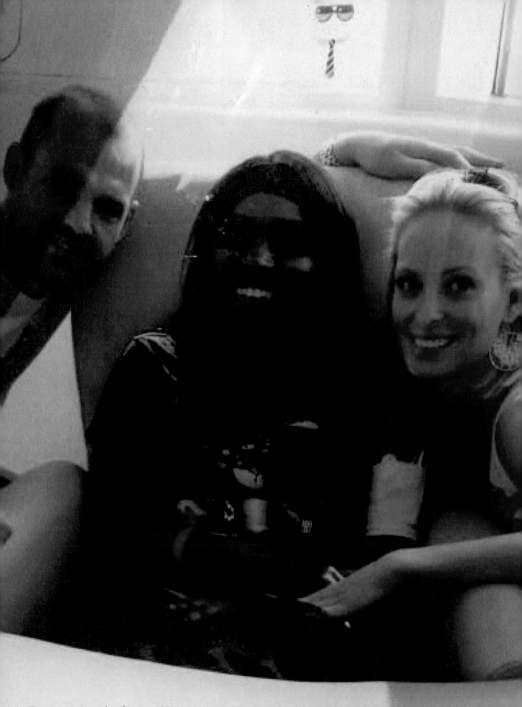

Danny Murphy | Myself in hospital [mid chemo & wig] | Joanna Taylor Murphy

Amidst The Misery

There are a few perks to being an in-patient at this hospital. The **Teenage Cancer Trust** work tirelessly to raise funds and donations so that young cancer sufferers like myself can get some enjoyment amidst the misery of their treatment. Today I go to see Kylie Minouge LIVE in concert at the o2 Arena London; FOR FREE and I am in a VIP box, can you imagine, what a treat. It does at times take my mind off my situation and either way it is a fantastic and memorable experience. There are other cancer patients here too and I listen to their stories, some of them have been battling cancer for years.

I also get to meet a footballer and his wife; I can hardly speak as my drugs protocol is intense and effects my mental state in many ways. The footballer is from Fulham FC but he used to play for Tottenham Hotspurs though, which is my team. They visit me in my hospital room, both are lovely and friendly and she [Joanna] is so tactile and warm. I find out that she is a **CLIC Sargent** patron. I am grateful for their visit, they really brighten up my day.

Lastly I go to meet Paris Hilton she is launching her perfume "Can Can" in Selfridge's. I am given a VIP pass; she seems really down to earth. Her boyfriend is a guy from the band "Good Charlotte" he loves the fact that I am called Charlotte and so do I right now.

It is great that the hospital, the Teenage Cancer Trust and CLIC Sargent are able to give me the opportunity to meet these people and to get out. It really helps me to take my mind off my situation, and I am grateful for this.

2008 - 2009

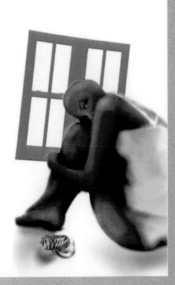

2 Steps Forward

Being in the chair means that a lot of my important muscles are not being stimulated. So a lot of simple tasks zap my energy. It is even exhausting standing in the shower, I bring a chair into the shower so I can sit instead of stand. This is difficult. I know that if I am to improve then I must get stronger and not rely on the wheelchair and other aids. However I am understandably weak from the treatment, stress, drugs and my condition; but on the flip side, the treatment is working so my condition is improving, therefore I must not get complacent.

I make a promise to myself that I will only use the chair if it is absolutely necessary. I know if I stick to this I will be pushing myself to progress by not taking the easy option. People actually stare at you more for walking differently than for being in a wheelchair, I think this is because people are less used to it.

I have now been in hospital a little over a month since my birthday. I am making slow but steady progress. My treatment is back on track, having been paused for a little while because I was mentally and physically in a bad condition. Things have now improved and I will be switching to another chemotherapy protocol. This schedule does not include the 'strong' intravenous Methotrexate, which is good for me in one way, but this protocol uses a different concoction of drugs so I will be on treatment for a longer period, but it will be considerably more manageable for me without the Methotrexate.

Still, I am dreading going back onto treatment. This new protocol still involves lumberpuntures, which will involve me having the same drug injected into my spinal and brain fluid, that shut my body down last time, therefore I am concerned and fearful.

I tell them I do not want to do this procedure anymore but they are adamant that it is an important part of my treatment. They tell me it will not effect me because the dose is minute compared to what I had intravenously. *I will later find out that this is a lie because it caused another girls body to shut down about a year later.* I have the lumber puncture whilst all the time worrying I am going to relapse.

Two weeks have passed and I feel a lot more relaxed that things are going to go smoothly. I am now well enough to leave the hospital but I still need intensive daily physiotherapy to make sure I can cope with getting around the house. This means I can not go home yet because the NHS physiotherapy in my area can only see me twice a week.

As a result the hospital put me up in the 5 star hotel across the road, it is lovely and my breakfast and dinner are paid for. Everyday I go over to the hospital for my physiotherapy, and then back to the hotel or sometimes I sightsee around central London.

It is now time for me to go home. The occupational therapists have checked to ensure the house and I have all the necessary equipment for me to get around ok.

I get home and it is an immediate reality check of how hard things are going to be. It becomes apparent to me that the doctors do not truly know what my future will be concerning my walking. I am just another patient so the goal is to cure the cancer by any means. I feel that they are not interested in my quality of life.

I hold quality of life high up there with things most important to me. The thing is the treatment I received is a one size fits all. The problem with that is when this treatment does not fit, there is not an alternative; which is what is happening in my case and I am rapidly getting disillusioned and loosing faith in the system.

Now I am out of hospital I feel it is pretty much out of sight out of mind. The NHS see me twice a week for physiotherapy and this is now to be reduced to once a week. I don't even feel the benefit from what they do with me. Am I sounding bitter and twisted? I don't know I'm just expressing how I feel about the situation right now. I'm 18 years old, I'm past halfway through my chemotherapy treatment. I've spent the best part of the last 6 months in hospital, I've lost my hair, walking is difficult, the drugs I take zap my energy and I feel that now that I am out of hospital I am not receiving as much support from the NHS as I feel I require [exhale]. So I've decided to get myself a personal trainer so I can boost my fitness levels. I progress a lot and gain some strength back.

My cousin Max is getting wed today and I am able to walk unaided but slowly. He sees me outside the church and starts crying tears of joy. I feel proud knowing I set myself a goal and have achieved it; even though my walking style is far from how I want it to be, I have still come so far.

Things are going well and I have not been admitted to hospital for weeks maybe months. Then in February 2009 I am admitted to my local hospital with a bad viral infection. The staff on the children's ward don't want me there because I am 18, however at my London hospital I am classed as a young person so this means the local hospital must keep me in their children's ward.

It is an uncomfortable stay feeling as if I am unwelcome on the ward. Some of the staff know me and are ok but others are not nice. I have my own private room but the bathroom is shared. I am given a course of antibiotics to combat my viral infection and I settle in for my stay.

I become quite weak in hospital and my fitness quickly declines along with my balance. I can no longer walk in a straight line and I am finding it hard to use my core muscles. It is like everything I have worked so hard to build over the previous months is just disappearing.

I finish my course of antibiotics and I am able to go home. My everyday routines have become much harder and I am no longer able to get around unaided. I quit the gym for a while as I am too unstable on my feet. If I am to recover from this relapse I will need a lot more physiotherapy than my current NHS offering of once a week.

I am fortunate and extremely blessed [*although I do not fully appreciate it at the time*] and my parents are able to pay for all of my rehabilitation treatments. *If it wasn't for them paying for all the things that give me hope, I may have given up a long time ago or even still be in a wheelchair!*

Don't get me wrong I am grateful for all the NHS have done for me, truly I am, but it is like there is not enough time or thought dedicated to my case. I have to do a lot of my own research and rely on the recommendations of others to get myself to where I am today.

Apart from the physiotherapy and speech therapy, no effort has been made to provide me with the knowledge of what has happened to me. I have seen a neurologist who says he has not seen such a severe case of immobility before caused as a reaction to a drug. He has seen something similar though, and the results he conveys are far from reassuring. He tells me one of the patients passed away and the other is still in a wheelchair.

This is a sure sign that I need to take action and to stop looking for outside reassurance. Relying on 'the system' will only take me so far. I get myself a private physiotherapist who I am able to see three times a week. I am only weeks away from my 19th birthday. I set a goal to be able to walk unaided by then. *I didn't really get to have a big celebration for my 18th*, my parents want this one to be more special.

Today is my 19th Birthday, April 2009 and thankfully I am at home.
It is definitely a special day for me. I take some of my good friends
in a limo *thanks Dad* from mine up to London. It takes us to a lovely
Caribbean restaurant hired out just for me with my own personal DJ
for the night. Unfortunately my walking is not where I had hoped for
it to be but there is great improvement, however I need crutches to get
around. Birthdays can be so stressful to celebrate but I don't know why
but having my friends around me today making me laugh is one of the
nicest feelings.

I am wearing a lace wig fitted to my head. However I am no longer
taking Doxorubicin; the drug that made my hair fall out is no longer
on my protocol. It is such a huge relief knowing that my hair is growing
back and it will no longer be falling out. That said, today is my birthday
and I want to look my best, but... from here-on in I have decided I
will no longer be wearing wigs. I am going to let my hair grow back
without fake hair; head-scarves and hats yes, wigs no.

I have decided I will no longer be wearing wigs. Head-scarves and hats yes, wigs no.

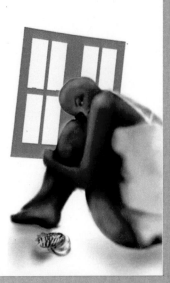

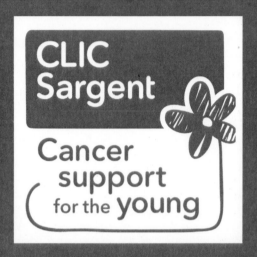

www.clicsargent.org.uk

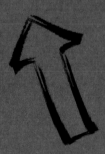

Lets Get Physical

It is Spring 2009 going into Summer and the texture of my new hair feels amazing, very different to the hair I had before I got ill. This is a good thing, a sign of better things to come *I hope, no I believe!*. Even though I still have a year of treatment remaining I am a step closer to the end, there is some light at the end of the tunnel. *When I am not awake I often dream of myself having long silky hair, it feels and seems so real.*

I think not wearing the wig has given me a push to start trying even harder and before I know it I am walking unaided. This is down to the concentrated effort I have been making on all fronts; the physiotherapy and gym sessions, the water intake and positive attitude.

I introduce my physiotherapist to my trainer in the gym so she can give my gym instructor some tips and I can once again begin to work on my physical recovery.

I am improving my fitness but only so far because the chemotherapy treatment knocks me back. I say knocks me back, it takes a lot out of me; the drugs effect my energy levels *at best*, and of course there can be other side effects.

Currently I have this dreadful constant pain in my left arm, I think I have pulled a muscle. It is so bad I need to have it strapped up on occasions, which helps a little. It has however become really weak and I can barely lift it, when I do lift it, it just drops back down. Not this again!

I mention the pain to my consultant at my check up and it is noted. Pain killers do offer some relief but no cure. I'm starting to think it is more serious than just a muscular injury.

Weeks pass and the pain shows no signs of abating, soon it will be months. I speak to the consultant again, she prescribes a MRI scan for both my shoulders. The results are in and shock horror, I have "avascular necrosis" in both shoulders. This is a side effect from long-term steroid use.

I am afflicted with Avascular Necrosis because the blood supply is being cut off from my shoulder ball joint bones, this causes the bone to wear away, which then leaves me with an rough surface 'Avascular Necrosis' making it hard for my arm to operate to its full capacity. I am told that further deterioration will mean I require a shoulder replacement.

They try to avoid doing this operation on people who are as young as I am, because it needs to be repeated every 10 years or so. I am told in the strictest terms to rest my arms and not to do any lifting or reaching. They tell me if I follow this advice it *should* reduce the need for me to have a shoulder replacement.

So I take the medical advice, I barely pick things up or put any weight through my arms. However it feels like things are getting worse. My arms are even weaker and I can barely lift up my left arm. The pain is constant causing me to believe I will need the shoulder operation before my treatment is finished.

They try to avoid doing this operation on people who are as young as I am, because it needs to be repeated every 10 years or so.

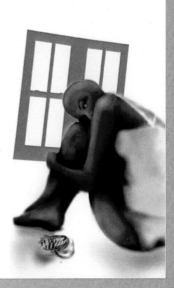

TEENAGE
CANCER
TRUST
CHALLENGING
CANCER
TOGETHER

Up & Running

I am still at home. My arm is still killing me. I am still determined to be positive about my recovery. My gym sessions have been limited because of my arm. However overall I am feeling ok within myself, so much so I have decided to resume my driving lessons. I already know how to drive manually but had to cancel my test when I became ill.

Alas my arm is too weak and I do not have the full range of movement. Changing gears and turning the steering wheel are too difficult for me right now. I must therefore learn in an automatic AND get a steering ball for my steering wheel.

I am upset about this because I know how to drive and now I have to go for an easy option. This option will enable me to drive now 'with a steering ball' but to drive unaided I will have to do a retest, which sucks. The good thing is that I will finally be getting on the road, which means a lot more freedom.

The day of my test arrives, it's an automatic and I have my steering ball, I pass. I feel like the luckiest person ever.

I can now drive myself and although I do not go out alone at first, the feeling of freedom and more significantly, 'accomplishment' are overwhelming. I also notice that driving starts to improve my arms movement. That's interesting, I make a conscious decision to start training my arms despite what I have been told about resting them.

I continue to train and my arm range continues to improve. I still avoid putting weight through them though as my shoulders are still in constant pain. In fact I am quite accustomed to the pain, I think I am learning to block it out.

I think I can avoid having an operation; if I do not express just how much pain I am in then they may not operate at this time. I do not highlight the pain anymore and I continue to exercise. *If I carry on this way I believe my arms will continue to improve at a slow but steady pace.*

People often say that you should look at the positive in every situation, so that's what I am doing. I am taken off the steroids because they caused my avascular necrosis. The consultants prefer I stay on the steroids because the play such a huge role in my cancer treatment. For me however, I am pleased because of all the horrible side effects I have had to endure over the past 12-18 months.

Stopping the steroid course makes such a positive difference to me. I feel and look more like myself again. My mind is clearer and my food obsession is abating. My food portions are now nearly half the size of before. All the extra weight I gained literally falls off. I still have the round chemotherapy face, caused from all the medication, but I am able to look in the mirror again without wanting to cry.

Things are looking up. I am back at home now and every time I face a new problem I can proudly say I don't let it keep me down, instead I search for a solution. I begin seeing a Kinesiologist who has also trained in many other alternative therapies, I really benefit from our sessions. She can also tell what is good and bad for the body and if anything is lacking in the body.

Her objective is to help me maintain a healthy mind and body inside and out. This is slightly different to the hospitals objective which is to kill the cancer. I believe working with them both will help me heal in the most efficient way. My consultant does not agree with what I am doing but it's my body and this approach just feels right.

*Stopping the steroid course makes
such a positive difference to me.
I feel and look more like myself
again.*

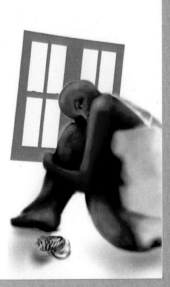

Which way do I go?
One is the hospitals alone
The other is unknown...

Crossroads

I wake up and I am at home which before my diagnosis was neither here nor there; but now waking up at home is always a good start to the day because it means I am not in hospital as I have often been these past 20 months.

Today my friend Drew is visiting and we are eating pizza. For some unknown reason my heart is beating very quickly. I am not stressed or excited so why is my heart beating so quickly? This feels weird.

I let my mum know what is going on and she calls the ambulance. Whilst we wait for the paramedics the palpitations abate and my heart beat settles so that by the time they arrive the issue has resolved itself; I am ok, but it was not a nice experience.

Today is the first time I drive my own car and all is well so far. However it seems I have spoken too soon. My heart is going really fast, the palpitations have returned and I am really hot. My hair is a hot mess so I'm not taking my hat off, I call for an ambulance... I am becoming too hot...

I must have passed out for what feels like minutes but could have been seconds I can't tell, however I feel better now. The ambulance is here but my heartbeat has returned to normal and so has my body temperature so there is not a thing they can do for me but take me home. I leave my car there and pick it up in the morning.

They say things come in threes, well I'm off to the restaurant with my friend. We order and as I drink this cola with my extra spicy hot food my heart starts going fast again. So much so that I ask Drew to drive. We leave and head back picking up Drew's mum on the way. I'm feeling hot again, my heart is beating all irregular...

I must have passed out again, I am now coming around, it's all hazy but Drew and his mum are very concerned and are doing their best to make me feel comfortable. It is working, I feel relaxed again and my body temperature is normalised. I am thankful that I am in safe hands.

Today I have a double physiotherapist session, well it's actually two single ones, one after another making it a double. The first single is with my NHS physiotherapist and the second with the private physio my parents are paying for. I complete both sessions but my heart starts 'going all irregular' again. Mum calls the ambulance. They are here and the paramedic asks me to lie on the floor with my legs elevated. My palpitations are detectable and my heart is beating so fast that the machine can not even take a reading.

I am rushed to the hospital, flashing blue lights and all. I am taken through to A&E and given a drug to slow down my heart rate. Everyone around me seems shocked at how I manage to remain so calm. I know if I panic it will just add more stress to my already strained heart.

They carry out several ECG'S [Electro Cardio Grams] but can not work out what is causing my palpitations. They want to put me on 'beater blockers' i.e. medication to control the heart rate. After my recent history with drugs and pills I feel I should read up on the possible side effects and that's what I do.

What's it say here? The nervous system can be effected, this does not sound too good. They discharge me with the medication and dosage instructions.

I feel I need a second opinion. I visit my kinesologist and show her the pills. When she checks my body she can not see anything wrong with the heart.

I start to look back on the four occasions I experienced the palpitations to see if I can find any common denominator. Caffeine, hot baths, and spicy food are all possible suspects you can also add 'emotional state' to that list. This is now a dilemma. My kinesologist has advised me of all the side affects taking the pills may cause, but my doctors have prescribed them suggesting they will cure the issue, thus implying if I do not take them that something bad will happen to my heart in the future. I have reached a crossroads, shall I follow the doctors blindly or shall I make my own decision based on my experiences and all the information I have at my disposal?

WHAT'S WORSE THAN HAVING LEUKAEMIA?

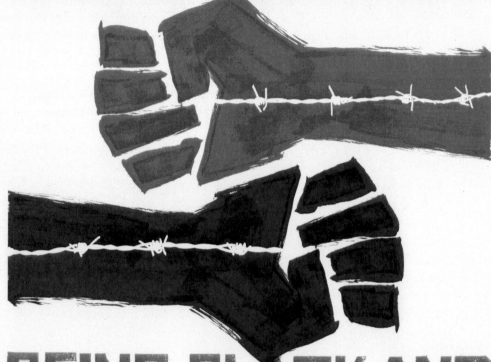

BEING BLACK AND HAVING LEUKAEMIA.

IT'S SHOCKING BUT IT'S TRUE. YOUR CHANCES OF FINDING A LIFE-SAVING BONE MARROW DONOR ARE MUCH WORSE IF YOU'RE BLACK – BECAUSE THERE ARE 24 TIMES MORE WHITE PEOPLE THAN BLACK PEOPLE ON UK BONE MARROW REGISTERS. TO CHANGE THIS, WE URGENTLY NEED MORE BLACK AND MIXED-RACE PEOPLE TO JOIN THE BONE MARROW REGISTER. JOIN OUR FIGHT TODAY – VISIT ACLT.ORG AND SEE JUST HOW EASY IT IS TO SAVE SOMEONE'S LIFE.

UNITE TO FIGHT LEUKAEMIA   aclt.org

The End Is Nigh

It is approaching the end of 2009 and I am about 5 months away from finishing my treatment. I am exhausted and quite fed up that every time I build up my energy and walking it is knocked right back down by the chemotherapy. One of the drugs I am on Vincristine, has me waking up crying because my whole body is pulsating with pain.

I tell my kinesologist about how I am feeling and I give her a list of everything I am still taking. I only take one of the drugs 'Vincristine' intravenously the rest are oral. I still have 5 months remaining before the Vincristine course ends.

The kinesologist suggests that this drug may be having an effect on my nervous system. This might explain why every time I take Vincristine I get set backs.

Time to do some more reading and research. Is there a possibility that Vincristine is causing my relapses. All the evidence I uncover suggests this is likely to be the case. I mention this to my consultant at my next check up. I am actually shocked to discover she is fully aware of the facts yet neglected to tell me. Her words imply that 'the priority is to cure the cancer irrespective of the side effects as we believe that the side effects are an acceptable consequence'

IMPORTANT: *What I do next is what I feel is right for me and I will never try to persuade people to follow in my footsteps unless they feel it is what is right for them.*

I decide to stop taking Vincristine 5 months before I am prescribed to. My consultant thinks this is an erroneous decision that may negatively effect the results of my treatment.

I feel it is the right choice and instantly I feel like a weight has been lifted from my shoulders. I decide not to lament on my choice but to continue with my recovery focusing on my walking.

Now that I have dropped Vincristine from my drugs protocol I only have oral pills on my schedule and nothing directly into my blood stream. One of the medicines I still take is called Macaptapurin, one of the instructions is 'No Milk' a few hours before or after taking the pill. Luckily I don't even like milk so ordinarily this would not be a problem but that does not stop me from craving milk. I think the fact that it is forbidden just adds to my desire. Funny how the mind can play tricks on you sometimes.

2010 - 2012

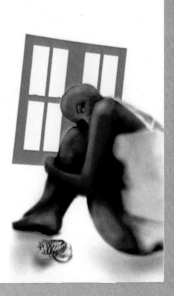

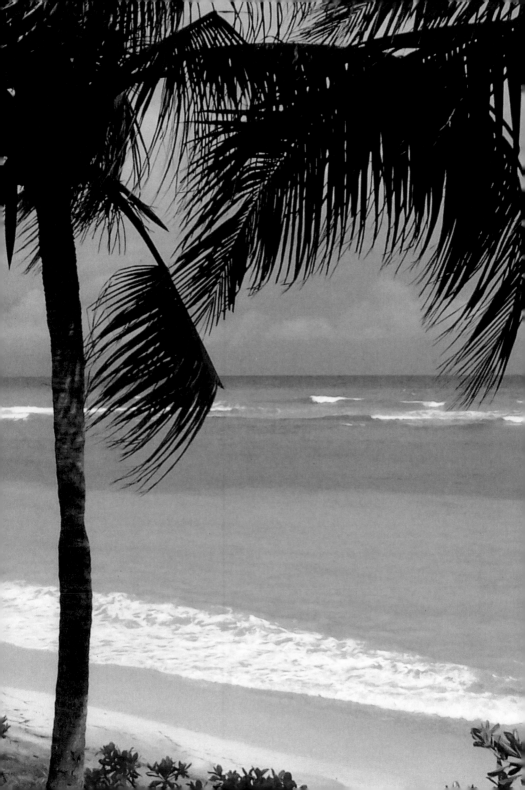

Land Of Milk & Honey

I am in the last months of treatment, I am allowed to go on holiday so I go to Jamaica, which has an amazing effect on my body. I stay with both sets of my grandparents; and I am spoilt with love and attention; in addition the abundance of fresh food and sun do wonders for my body and mind. Everything is going smoothly, I don't have to worry about the dreadful side effects I suffered when taking Vincristine. I turn 20 on the 19th April 2010, eleven days away from the end of my chemotherapy treatment.

It is the 30th of April 2010 and I have finally finished my treatment. I am so happy. I know things are only going to be uphill from here. I'm not feeling a big celebration so I am not going to make a big deal of it.

Ironically on this, one of the most significant days of my treatment; I get some unrelated bad news. My great grandma, Aunty Darrell has passed away. Is it unrelated? I am not sure I just have a very strong feeling and in this moment I envision her to be my guardian angel, I do not believe in coincidences, everything happens for a reason. I attend the funeral in Jamaica accompanied by Mum, my two aunts and two cousins.

I know that even though my treatment is now over it is still going to take some time before I feel normal again. I spend most of my time studying and trying to rebuild my body again. I slowly regain a good amount of strength but my round chemo face is taking longer to go back down. My walking is getting better if at a very slow pace and if I am being honest with myself, at this rate it could take years before I can walk properly. This is NOT a motivating prospect, however during the hell of the past few years I have acquired key skills, one of which is positive thinking and I am learning how powerful the mind can be. I tell myself that the journey to walking properly will be a long one but I will never give up working towards my goal, no matter how long it takes. *This is important because it is hard to stay motivated when you are not seeing much improvement for your endeavours. This is when your mind needs to be strong, to enable you to focus and not to lose hope no matter how arduous the journey may be. It is also widely believed that your positive thoughts translate into positive energy which in cases of recovery can effect positive physical results far beyond those expected.*

Although my chemotherapy treatment has concluded I continue to be monitored by the hospital. I have a schedule of regular check ups at 6 week intervals. Other than this my days are mainly spent at home educating myself or in the gym training. I go out with friends to eat or even just sit in the party booths when it is someone's birthday. I also spend a lot of time with my close and extended family and with my friends, sometimes venturing to the cinema. Although to be honest... I am so self-conscious about how I look as a result of the past two years, that staying in is my preferred option.

*It is believed that your positive
thoughts translate into positive
energy which in cases of recovery
can effect positive physical results.*

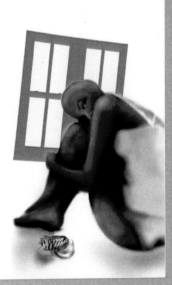

My body does not work as well as it did prior to the cancer even though the cancer has now gone.

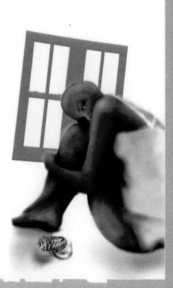

The New Normal

It is over two years since my first diagnosis and my chemotherapy treatment ended a few months back, yet it feels a little like the reality of cancer is only now sinking in. It is like there are three realities that you have to come to terms with. One is the actual affliction and what that does to your body. The second is the effect the chemo has on your mind and body. Finally there is the reality that now that the treatment is finished my body has not returned to the condition it was in prior to my diagnosis. It does not go back to normal. Instead there is a new normal and it is not an improved version but the opposite. My body does not work as well as it did prior to the cancer even though it has now gone.

Two patients who I was closest to on my journey both pass away and this really shocks me. Until now I have been reluctant to be seen by the world because I fear being judged. This shocking news acts as a catalyst for me. I tell myself I am being selfish, at least I am still here and at least my friends and family have not lost me. I must stop worrying about what others think because I am lucky to still be here... I must get on with life.

I start to apply for jobs and continue networking, I take a few interviews but I do not get hired. I will not let the rejections get me down because it is all experience; plus I make some amazing new connections along the way.

I continue to ease myself 'back into society'. Aunt Lizzie is to be married in Jamaica and I am to be one of the bridesmaids. I help her with some of the planning and it gives me something to look forward to. It also means I will be returning to Jamaica, I benefited greatly from my previous trip and I am excited to be returning so soon.

The wedding is amazing and I even manage to walk down the isle in heels. This is one of my favourite trips to Jamaica as my family is united around the event with attendees converging from all over the place; UK, USA, Canada and Jamaica, some I have not seen in ages others I have not met in person before. It is so much fun. I am actually feeling more like my old self. The vibe out here is just crazy and the energy levels are 100. Good food, good music and good people.

Time to come home to the UK, my spirits are high from my holiday and I continue with my recovery schedule. I have also fallen in love with dancehall music; a style of reggae. There is one dancehall website in particular that I visit regularly and the owner is based here in the UK, I reach out to him. The response is positive and I start to help them with the social media side and as a result I begin to forge links with many people in the industry.

I don't even think he knows how grateful I am for the opportunity because from this platform I am able to rebuild my confidence.

Sprinkled amongst all this 'life' activity are my hospital check up visits. I have a new consultant and clinical nurse and they are a great team. They are 'on it' anything I need help with they are quick to assist.

I am still adapting to walking, whilst continuing with my long term objective of being able to walk as before or as close to. My hips are hurting, it feels similar to the shoulder pain I experienced from the avascular necrosis.

In my head I am thinking it can't possibly be avascular necrosis as I have been off steroids a few years now and the steroids were identified as the cause last time. However to be sure I am taken for a MRI scan on my hips.

My worst fears are confirmed I have avascular necrosis in both of my hips. *It was probably there at the same time as when I had found it in my shoulders but I was not walking much then nor in the same way so I had not felt any discomfort previously.*

The pain is horrible even with my high pain threshold. The doctors advise me once again to just rest and not do too much on my legs, no jumping and limited exercise, *but we've been here before and we know better don't we?*

My right hip hurts a lot more than my left, and it often just gives way. This is making me feel very unsteady on my feet. I am fearful of putting too much weight through the right leg and as a result I am putting extra pressure on my left leg to compensate.

I have stopped my personal training at the gym and instead I am doing more workouts from home plus physiotherapy. I also get a yoga instructor who comes here to the house and teaches Mum also.

I am studying the law of attraction amongst other things and I see how I might have attracted certain things into my life over time. The mind is all so powerful and effects the body; although this works both ways, so a negative mind-set can have a negative effect on the body.

2012 - 2014

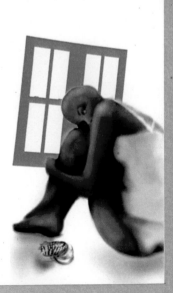

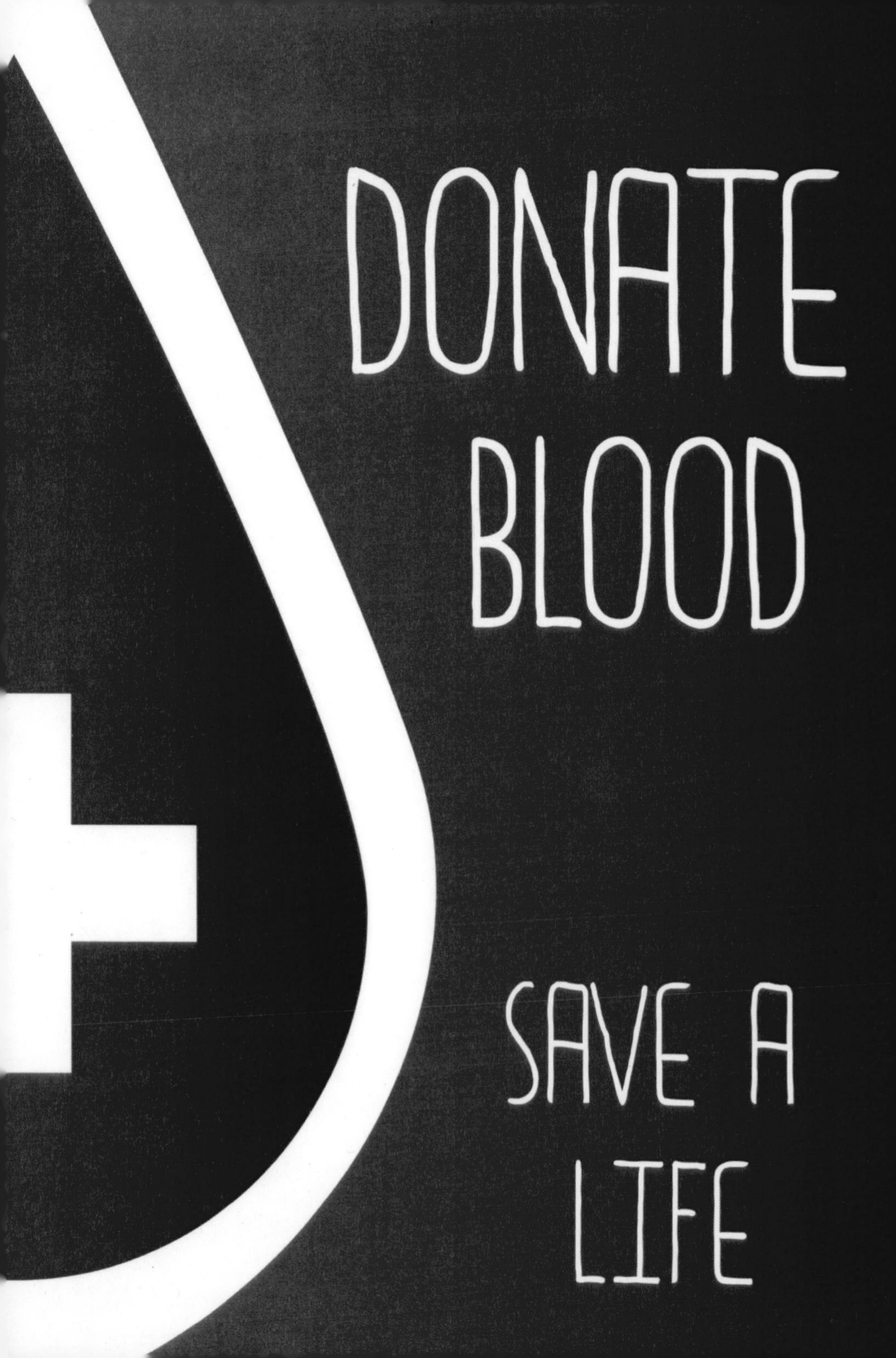
DONATE
BLOOD
SAVE A
LIFE

Thank you

When I was diagnosed with cancer back in 2007 I was 17. My chemo started within months and by the time I was 18 I was fully into my treatment schedule. As a teenage cancer sufferer I was given many wonderful treats by charities who support hospitals, sufferers and carers. **The Teenage Cancer Trust** were great and also **Dreams Come True**; who make wishes come true for under 21's especially those with life threatening conditions.

In 2012 I made a wish via the Dreams Come True charity; I wished for a trip to New York, including shopping spree. However at that time my body was in a bad way, it had shut down at times and I was experiencing many uncomfortable side effects. So I put off completing the dream until I was in a better condition to go. Well here we are in 2013 and I am in way much better condition than I was back then. Time to complete that application and get my wish, so I do just that. I have to wait a little, as there are quite a few people who have a much greater need for their wish than me. I'm actually recovering now, others are currently having to experience what I did back then or worse; so their need is understandably greater than mine.

The wait is over and today my wish will be fulfilled. As part of my wish I am allowed to take one person with me for free. There is only really one candidate for that spot and that is Mum. She has been on this journey with me every step of the way and never complains, she is my rock and friend and I could not have got through this without her support. She picks me up, she shares my tears then wipes them away, we continually laugh along the way and there are so many great if not painful memories. She deserves this trip as much as I need it.

I am currently reading a book called "The Magic" by Rhonda Byrnes who also wrote "The Secret" another great book. Rhonda talks about daily activities, positivity and gratitude. This is a perfect opportunity to execute the daily activities, as suggested in the book. I am grateful and thankful for all my mum has done for me so she is the perfect person to share my wish with.

So off we go. We arrive at the airport and our seats get upgraded on the plane, we board and enjoy a pleasant flight. We land and I receive a text saying out driver is waiting for us. Driver AND limousine... talk about travel in style. He drives us to this amazing hotel that looks more like something out of the movies. We are in the heart of the city, the staff are great and we want for nothing.

Time to get out and about, we eat out at lots of restaurants and all the food we choose is lovely and fresh. We go shopping, the deals are amazing out here. Best of all my energy and stamina are running at 100% I feel great. What a great trip thank you Dreams Come True for such a wonderful experience. I don't want to leave, but alas we must come home.

dreams come true
Bringing joy to terminally and seriously ill children

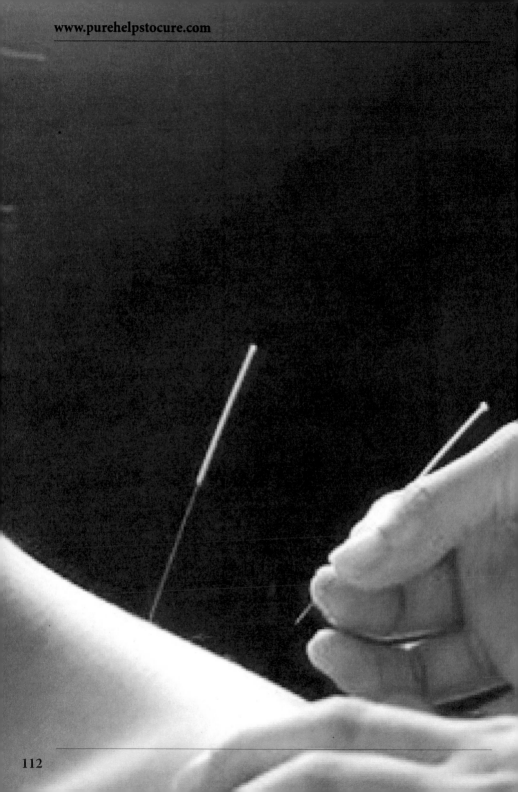

Healing Hands

I am still buzzing after my amazing Dreams Comes True New York shopping trip, I am in a totally new frame of mind. I think back to how I was able to avoid having a shoulder replacement; I tell myself it is in my power to improve my hips and thus avoid a hip replacement.

I have been following the instructions given to me by my doctor and admittedly my hips have not worsened as a result but nothing has improved either. I am in my early twenties and I can not imagine the rest of my life being restricted because of my hips. Time to take action like I did with the shoulders and my arm.

I up my yoga sessions and I start back at the gym with a new personal trainer who my brother has introduced me to. I continue with my physiotherapy. I am progressing I can actually feel a physical improvement, which is very motivating.

Mum and Dad have been house hunting for some time. They have found somewhere and we are moving from my childhood home, which I have lived in since I was 8 years old. Despite this connection I am actually glad to leave as there are too many memories relating to my illness. Moving to the new house motivates me more.

My aunt introduces me to an acupuncturist and this man is good. He uses herbs, massage and acupuncture. The chemotherapy had a long lasting effect on my insides but he is able to help redress the damage with herbs which I add water to and drink every morning and night. He advises me to change my sleeping position, and this along with the acupuncture makes a big difference. The massages he gives are great for loosening the body and helping me to relax.

I add a chiropractor team to my ever growing list of support, they work wonders with aligning my body. Although it seems I will have to let the chiropractor go as these things are not cheap. However my motto is if you are seeing results don't stop. Therefore I have a dilemma as the chiropractor is good for me.

2015

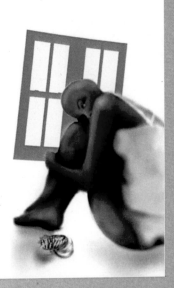

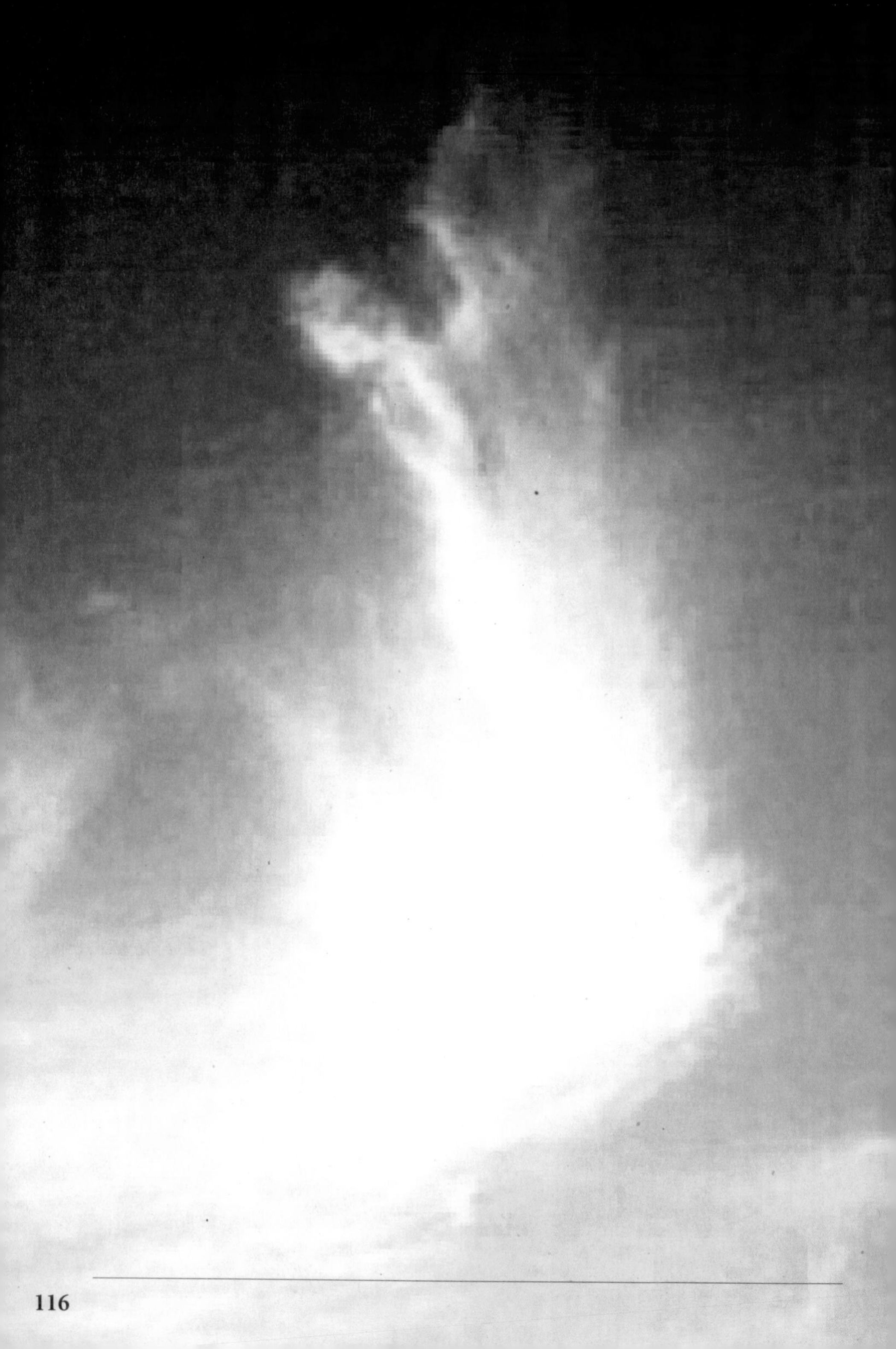

Saint Michael

Thankfully or unfortunately I don't really know which, but either way I do not have any previous cancer experiences to call upon. If you are fortunate you only get cancer once but that means you don't know what to expect. For me it was tough but now I am in recovery the 'new normal' is less difficult than cancer itself, but it is difficult nevertheless.

Chemo finished in August 2010, last year 2014 proved to be a good year for both my physical and mental development. However it is now 2015 and I am feeling like I may have reached my peak. I feel like I am just coasting along at the same stage and that nothing is really getting any better than the year before.

In life you have to take the steps to move forwards but sometimes things can happen for a reason just when you need them. As part of my 'new normal' I have joined a book club "Soul Sisters". The group meet once every month or so and we review positive and motivational books. We have read many great books but one of my current favourites is "The Slight Edge".

This book really speaks out to me at a time in my life when I feel a bit lost. It gives me a whole new perspective of how I need to look at lifes situations and how I should add lots of new positive habits to my daily routine. I can work with this philosophy, lets give it a try. One of the habits I add to my daily routine is an early morning chat with my dad before he leaves for work. It helps and turns out to be a nice start to the day for me.

Today I sit down with him and explain how I feel stuck with my walking or should I say 'my not walking properly'. I tell him that I have become everyone's little project, and how I am bombarded with countless suggestions and numerous "try this and try thats" yet I am not seeing any positive results. I tell him that I just don't know what to do anymore. I can see by the look in his eyes that he wants to help but does not know how.

A few days have passed since I spoke to my dad about my latest walking issues yet it seems he has been busy during that time. He's here with someone called Michael, Dad says he has brought Michael here to give me some advice and explains to me that he thought long and hard about what I had said earlier and that he thinks this man Michael may be able to help.

After the initial introductions Michael studies my walking both in real-time and he also watches a previously recorded video of me walking. After this he tells me that he believes he can help me. He then proceeds to describe my walking issues with such accuracy you'd think he is experiencing the issues himself. What he says is a combination of what every different person I have worked with over the past few years has told to me but rolled into one detailed explanation. We arrange our next session and our alliance begins.

The first session is a combination of tests to see what my limitations are; it is shocking how much we discover in only a few hours. Michael says that the reason I have become so stuck with my walk and unable to improve any further is because I have created my current walking pattern based on a fear of falling over; and as a result I have been using all the wrong muscles, which has given me this unbalanced and sometimes painful walking pattern.

It is then that he tells me that he is willing to see me a few evenings each week. He explains that I will have to go back to basics and this will mean taking some backward steps so that I can move forwards. We begin the regular sessions and my brother is on hand most evenings for practical and emotional support.

I really do have to go back to basics; Michael suggests I get a walking frame to assist. He says this will eliminate my fear of falling thus enabling me to perfect my walking pattern using the correct muscles. Going to get the frame from the shop feels horrible, I thought I'd done with walking aids. Michael advises I limit the weight I put through my arms when using the frame and just use it as a "safety net".

Mum, Dad and I are returning to Jamaica end of August 2015; this is just over two weeks away. Michael is totally convinced I will be able to change my walk before we fly. This gives us 14 days or so. I am happy with Michael and everything he is doing for me but I'm not sure about this time-line. Especially after the past few years where nothing has seemed to go to schedule.

No one and I mean NOT ANYONE has been able to help me improve at a fast rate over all these years. Before Michael came along I actually had a dream suggesting that I would be getting help from an unexpected source. It turns out Michael may just be that unexpected source. I continue to see Michael daily and my walking really improves.

It is time to leave for Jamaica and my walking pattern has really improved. Just a few key adjustments have helped the look and feel of my walk. I even began to feel my confidence returning and I can envision myself running again. This is perfect timing! I think to myself that I will use this trip as time to really embed what I have learned into my mind and body.

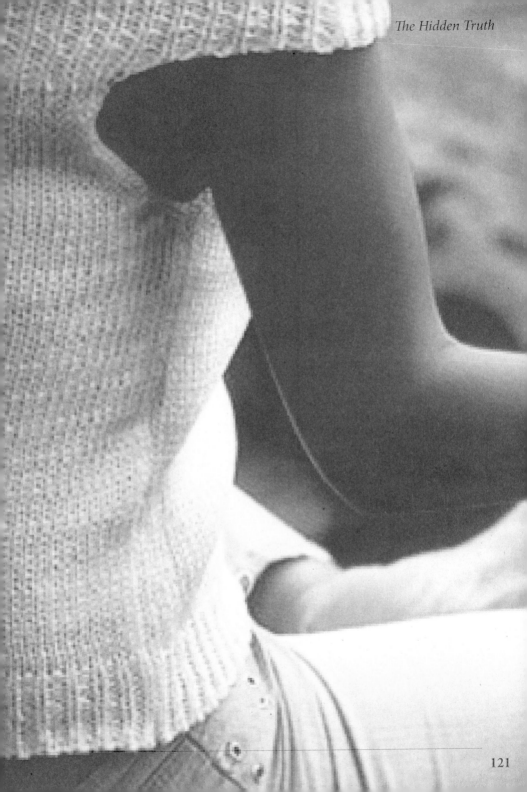

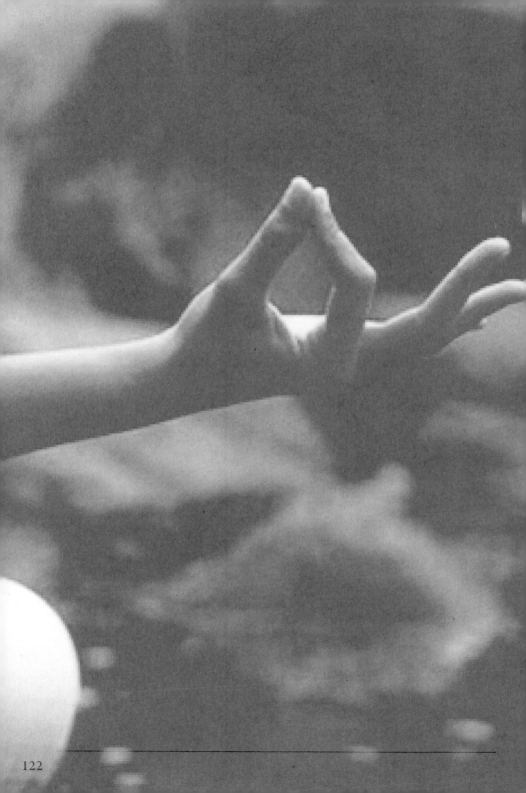

Paradise Revisited

I am really excited about this trip, I have an extra skip in my step, literally. I still need a little airport assistance and that upsets me a little but that's the reality. However this time I have the consolation that I'm in a much better condition than last time and I haven't even taken off yet. The flight is definitely my best aeroplane experience to date. The food is actually really nice and the time seems to just fly by, ah (I exhale)... the benefits of a nice relaxing flight.

We land in Jamaica and my body is tingling with 'energy' it's the only way I can describe how I feel, although 'uplifting' is another word that comes to mind. This can be due to a combination of factors; my improved walking, my expectations for the coming holiday and the new environment are all candidates for the reason I am feeling so amazing. I step out of the airport and breathe in the fresh air, I feel my entire body just relax. I am already feeling the benefits of this wonderful Island and I have not done a thing yet.

Everything about me just loves the Jamaican environment and it gives me the opportunity to spend time with my grandparents and sort out business ventures. I keep on top of my training, I don't want to regress. I spend a lot of my mornings with my dad on the Manchester golf course practicing my exercises, watching the sunrise, it is blissful. The grass makes exercising much easier and takes the pressure off my knees.

My walking and balance have improved I think I even look taller, because my posture is better. Today I am walking on the road whilst my mum films me. It is trickier on the road and challenges my balance.

Altogether in general I have much more energy and better fitness due to my daily exercise routine. Add to this the abundance of fresh food, relaxed atmosphere, wonderful weather and loving companions; and the apparent glow on my face makes more sense. My grandparents eat from the land and grow much of their own food so I get to taste paradise as well.

Most importantly I have a better state of mind, more positivity and more confidence. My family and friends have noticed the changes and are complimenting me on how well I look.

I think what I love most about Jamaica is that I never feel like I am being judged. The people who I know over here also talk freely so I always know where I stand with them. I will return to London tomorrow feeling refreshed and ready to move on to the next part of my training. Full of enthusiasm yet regret, I mean who wants to leave paradise!

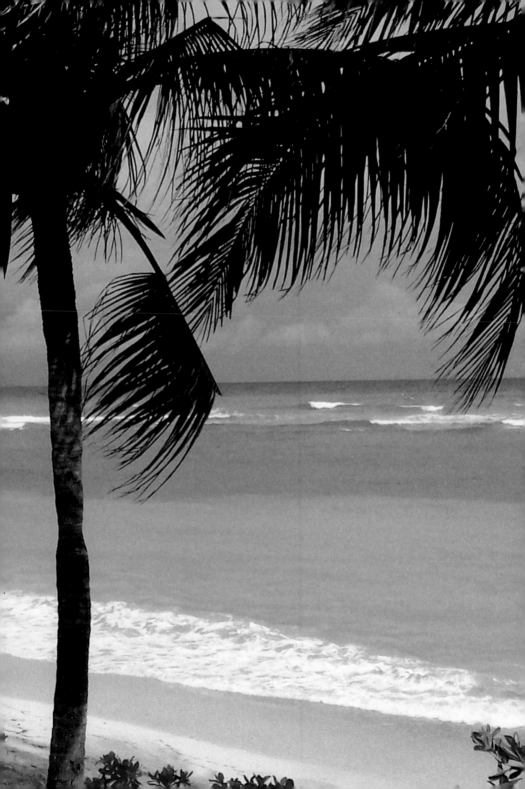

I have set up a website:
www.purehelpstocure.com
which gives tips and advice about
healthy living and natural healing.

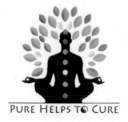

PURE HELPS TO CURE

Checking Out

I have returned from Jamaica and I am here in the UK. I have a neurologist appointment. I'm expecting to get some positive reinforcement as well as closure on what really happened all those years ago. When I ask the neurologist to explain and discuss my case he is very evasive, I think this is slightly odd.

I list the side effects that I am still suffering from daily. One of them is becoming more apparent and that is yawning plus my lack of concentration when listening to people. He tells me this has always been there but it is probably more noticeable because I am doing more and more things.

He then carries out some standard tests to do with movement, strength and reflexes. He tells me my strength is really good but the issue is more to do with the cerebellum, which is the base of the brain. This is the same part of the brain that is effected when you drink alcohol, therefore things like my speech and co-ordination are effected.

I ask him if he thinks I can make a full recovery and he says after five years most people have peaked, and are unlikely to improve any further after such an amount of time. For me it has been seven years so…(basically no). He refers me to the rehabilitation team and leaves it at that.

Please excuse my language but I know what he is telling me is complete bullshit! In the last few weeks alone I have already seen improvement in my coordination through working with 'Saint Michael'. *I'm not going to lie, what the neurologist says still hits a nerve [no pun intended], to this day.* I am about to turn 25 that's FIVE years in remission and honestly between you and me, all those years ago I thought I would be actually running sprints by now.

This neurologist can surely do with a lesson in positive reinforcement skills or maybe he is having a bad day. Either way it makes me understand why some people can give up especially when you have trained professionals stamping all over 'your hope'. You have to be really strong minded because no matter how positive you are it can be a challenge to ignore negativity in any form. That's exactly what it is, negative information, not fact because actually I am still improving.

The next time I see my consultant I tell him what happened at the neurologist session. He gives me positive feedback saying "I should be proud of myself because I never give up". I am sad as this is my last meeting with the consultant and my clinical nurse. They have helped me the most and are by far my favourite, I will miss their support, care and advice.

I am now too old to be going to the young persons clinic and I am told I will be moving to the next steps clinic in 2016. I am also told that my fertility may be effected as a result of the chemo. I didn't realise but my mum tells me this was explained to me years ago when I was originally diagnosed. Apparently there is even a chance I may start my menopause early. The advice is to have kids sooner rather than later. Well for now this is not on the horizon so I won't bother putting too much thought to it.

It has been approximately one month since I saw my neurologist and clinical nurse for the last time. Today I am to be assessed as prearranged by 'the' rehabilitation team; consisting of a doctor, nurse, occupational therapist, speech therapist and physiotherapist. I tell them everything I have done over the years and what I am doing to rehabilitate myself and also what things I want to improve.

They seem to think I have done a real great job so far and it seems like I am on the right track with my current trainer so they do not think they will be able to add anything. The physiotherapist is very impressed with my strength and there seems to be only ONE movement that indicates I have a weakness; all the rest are ok.

My speech is classed as fine. I have not had any speech therapy for years I just sing a lot and talk a lot (lol), which seems to have helped. One thing I dislike is my new low voice especially since it used to be quite squeaky hence why one of my good friends calls me squeaks. The speech therapists do some tests and I am still able to reach some high notes. She thinks I may be using the wrong muscle to talk with and suggests I talk from my chest and get a voice coach.

This assessment has been so positive, I have been told for once to continue with what I am doing as it seems to be working and I may also have a solution to help my voice. This is important to me because my voice plays a huge part in how I feel about myself and my confidence can be effected because I worry that people can't understand me when I talk.

I'd love to have finished this book saying I can run but not just yet.
I do know I am on the way and my brother has been amazing and
has being doing a lot of research into the body and how it should
be. He is helping me realign my body as he noticed that I have been
overloading on the right side and my posture has been wrong. He
is helping me wake up muscles, which have been sleeping for seven
years because I have been using the wrong muscles. Saint Michael
is still here helping me with technique, coordination and body
conditioning.

My brother Jason and 'Saint Michael' as a team have been great and
without both of their input I know I wouldn't have made the amazing
progress, which I have already made. I am truly thankful for their
time, research and effort, which they have put in to helping me. Mum
and Dad have been selfless and I dare not even imagine how much
more difficult and at times impossible this situation would have been
without them.

I am glad I have been able to share my story with you and it is nice
to see so many other people sharing their journeys lately. A lot of the
time we just hear about people who lose their lives from cancer or
survive it. I wanted to also share the mental and physical conditions
that these drugs can induce because it should not be hidden.

I have set up a website called www.purehelpstocure.com which gives
tips and advice about healthy living and natural healing, please feel
free to visit, and please do not hesitate to drop me a line. I will try to
answer every message I get. I hope you get something positive from
my experience.

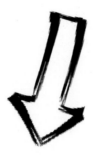

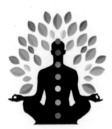

PURE HELPS TO CURE

www.purehelpstocure.com

Glossary & Tips

BLOOD TESTS – I remember before I got my pic line I had lots of cannula in my left hand, it got to a point where they found it hard to find my veins. My hand would be so sore and the skin even turned blue and bruised.

BLOOD TRANSFUSION - Taking in blood via a bag from a healthy person who has the same blood type as you. I had at least three transfusions and always felt quite energetic after.

BONE MARROW TEST – Taking some of the bone marrow to check for cancer cells. I was put to sleep for this procedure but when I came round I remember being very sore at the point from which they had extracted the marrow.

CT/CAT SCAN (Computerised Axial Tomography) – The purpose of this scan is to show a detailed picture of the body tissues. You lay flat on a bed, which slides in and out of a long cylinder shaped machine. You have to keep still and sometimes they inject a dye, which can give you a hot flush feeling. It's like a long dark tunnel, but it looks worse than the actual experience.

ECG (Electro Cardio Gram) - This measures the electrical activity of the heart. They put sticky sensors all over your chest, which are connected to a machine that records your heart readings. I had to get these quite regularly as chemotherapy can have an effect on the heart. When I was having bad palpitations I had to wear a mini one for a whole day, just my luck that my heart didn't even flutter that day [p.90-92].

LUMBER PUNCTURE – I would have this so they could check the fluid, which surrounded my brain and spinal cord. They would also inject me for chemo. After the procedure I would have to lay flat for a while so I could avoid headaches or dizzy spells. The first few times I had the lumber puncture I was put to sleep but when I woke up I would feel groggy and sore and very hungry from where I had to be nil by mouth. So I started to get them whilst I was awake and they would just numb the area rather than putting me to sleep. It felt weird because you could still feel the movement of what they were doing, and on a few occasions I got a sharp pain down my leg. The main reason I opted to do it this way was so I could eat more quickly afterwards plus it wouldn't be so sore because they seemed to take more care when I was under a local anaesthetic.

MRI SCAN (Magnetic Resonance Imaging) - Used to create an image of the inside of the body. This machine is extremely noisy they sometimes play music but you can barely hear it. You have to stay very still otherwise they have to repeat a section. This is most definitely my least favourite scan, and whichever part of the body they are scanning gets caged down. It's also feels claustrophobic because everything is very close to your face.

PET SCAN (Position Emission Tomography) – This scan shows you what the body tissues look like and how they are working. It is also used to determine which stage of cancer you have, if the treatment is working and to assist in deciding what the next treatment should be. They inject you with a warm liquid which may make you feel like you have wet yourself; every time I had this scan I always checked the bed when I got up because I thought I had.

PLATELET TRANSFUSION – Platelets are small cells in your blood, which help you form clots to stop bleeding. When my platelet count was low I had to have a transfusion; and like the blood transfusion this Platelet version also felt like it gave me extra energy afterwards.

ULTRASOUND – Where sound waves are used to build up a picture of the inside of the body. I had to get several of these done on my heart and liver, it does not hurt but can feel quite uncomfortable when they push down plus the jelly they use is really cold.

X-RAY- High energy rays taking pictures of the inside of the body. I have had countless over the years and still have to get one for my shoulders and hips once a year, to see if the avascular necrosis has worsened.

Complementary Therapies and Alternative Healing

Only use registered practitioners or people who you are referred to!

ACUPUNCTURE – This is a form of treatment using needles inserted along your meridian lines to help treat you. This is great and has helped to alleviate a lot of the ailments I have accrued as a result of my cancer treatment. Fist thing is first, does it hurt? Most needles you don't feel go in and others you can I guess. The needles are thinner than the average.

CHIROPRACTOR – This procedure helps to align the joints. I love it and feel great after a session; you will be shocked at what a chiropractor can help you with. You will definitely hear cracking sounds so if you are squeamish I do not recommend.

KINESIOLOGY – This is a holistic therapy, which works on your physical, emotional, psychological, nutritional and spiritual levels. This is great for finding out if your body is lacking in anything or has too much of something; they work a lot with energy.

MEDITATION AND VISUALISATION – This helped and helps me big time. I would visualise myself in my favourite place. Or when my mind is overflowing with questions I just meditate to clear it.

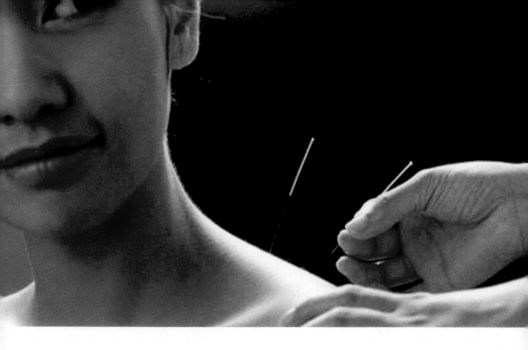

MASSAGE – I love massages they are great for relaxing tension and stress and just relaxing the body.

PRAYERS AND SPIRITUAL HEALING – I had a lot of people praying for me all over the world and I think all their positive vibes definitely played a role in keeping me positive. I also visited a few spiritual healers, which also boosted my energy. The jury is still out on whether these things are real; however either way I felt the positivity and believed so that alone can make a difference to your positive energy levels.

REIKI – Where energy is channelled into you to activate natural healing. There was a lovely man at the hospital who had lost his son to cancer and he would come round to give patients reiki. It would leave me feeling very calm and relaxed

REFLEXOLOGY – A system of massage performed on the hands, feet and head to treat illness. A lady also used to come round and do this in the hospital too, it felt lovely and relaxing.

My Diet

This is not a strict regime for you to follow but you can get an idea of what type of foods worked for me. Please feel free to contact me directly if you would like personalised dietary or nutritional advice. Visit www.purehelpstocure.com. I choose one from each section each day but you can mix and match as you wish.

Start the day with a small cup of warm lemon water or desirable herbal tea

Breakfast:
1. Oatmeal (almond milk) with raisins and flax-seeds
2. Quinoa and apple porridge
3. 2 eggs scrambled or boiled and avocado
4. Green smoothie
5. Fried egg sandwich with plantain (Cheat meal)
6. Ackee salt fish dumpling (Cheat meal)
7. Spinach, mushrooms, green bananas, avocado
8. Fresh mixed berries, (strawberries, blueberries, raspberries & blackberries)
9. Banana pancakes
10. Salt-fish Fritters & plantain

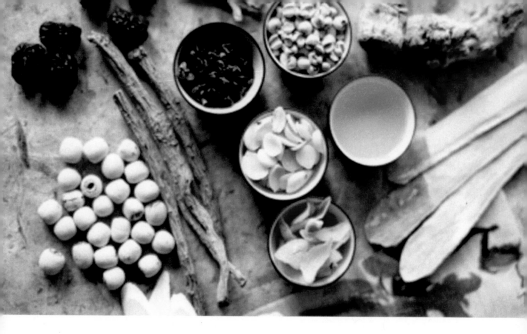

Lunch:
1. Wild Salmon fillet, butter-bean mash and veg
2. Ackee veg and wild rice
3. Tuna on sweet potato bake
4. Vegetable open pie
5. Fish with collie flower and broccoli creamed sweet potato
6. Beetroot burger and wedges
7. Prawn salad wraps
8. Chickpea and lentil burgers
9. Vegetable stir fry with spelt pasta
10. Sweet ginger Korean style mushrooms, Wild rice and salad

Drink: about 2 litres of water throughout the day
If I eat out or have any junk food, I tend to leave it until the weekends.

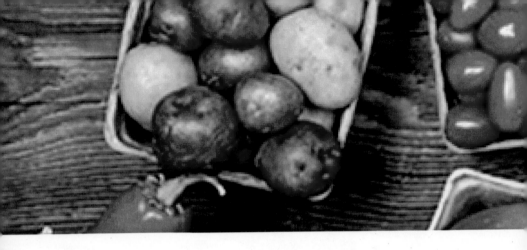

Dinner:
1. Super-food Salad – beetroot, sweet potato, avocado, quinoa, cucumber, spinach leaves and pumpkin seeds.
(add meat or fish if you like)
2. Lentil stew
3. Stew peas and rice or potato
4. Pea, carrot, bok choy and quinoa (add meat or fish if you like)
5. Soup (mushroom; vegetable; courgette; tomato &bell peppers)
6. Wild Salmon and vegetables
7. Courgette gratin and wedges
8. Lentil chilli con carni
9. Green Banana, Sea Bream and vegetables
10. Vegetable curry with sweet potato mash

Snacks:
1. Fresh fruit
2. Nuts
3. Humus and wholemeal pitta or cucumber sticks
4. Green banana chips
5. Olives

I like to have my lightest meal in the evening.

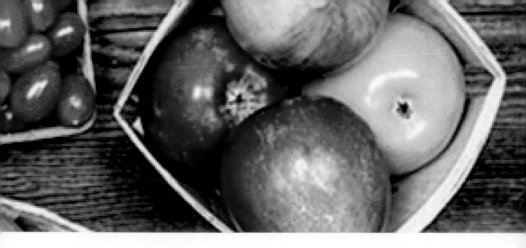

Desserts (in moderation):
1. Banana & chocolate cake
2. Dark Chocolate 70% coco
3. Dairy free ice cream
4. Baked fruit vegan tart crumbles
5. Sweet potato brownies

Drinks:
1. Spring water
2. Detox water (fresh fruit infused in water)
3. Homemade herbal teas (that way you can be sure of the ingredients)

Drink: about 2 litres of water through out the day (preferably spring)

General Tips:
>>> I like to have my lightest meal in the evening.
>>> As I am pescatarian trying to transition to vegan most meals are vegetable or fish based but you could use meat instead if you want.
>>> If I eat out or have any junk food, I tend to leave it till the weekends and work it off within the next day or two.

Family & Friends

I was really looking forward to this part of the book because my family and friends were a big part my journey. I cannot stress enough how important it is to have support and love from other people. I know it can be hard to not shut people out which is something I did at times; but people who care about you and make you laugh are important because when you are feeling down it is great to have people there to uplift you. I think I will begin with my immediate family, and like I said at the beginning of the book I felt that we lived quite a disconnected life before I got ill. We all just pretty much did our own thing, but right now we are definitely closer than ever. I think my illness may have really helped to highlight what is important and we are a tight unit. Plus the birth of both my beautiful nephews has been like a sign of better things to come.

Mum stopped working so she could care for me full time, she practically lived with me when I had to stay in hospital. No words alone can ever begin to describe how grateful and lucky I am for what she did for me. I then need to step back and take a look at my parents as a unit because I truly don't know where I would be today without them. They have paid thousands of pounds over the years for my rehabilitation, which I have consistently maintained since April 2008.

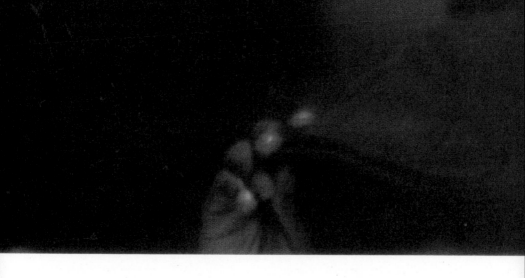

My brother and sister are the best siblings I can ever ask for. They have never treated me differently and they always keep it real. They are both loving caring siblings whom I have grown closer to and they have my back no matter what. I'm very lucky that my brother is now a Personal Trainer and is helping me get better week by week.

A lot of the time you actually see these kinds of situations break families up. Now I am not saying it hasn't been hard and testing on us because at times it has been difficult, but it has highlighted our strengths and shown how strong we can be through tough times.

My extended family have also been a great support to my family and myself. I am especially touched by those who joined me for Christmas 2007, to think people took time out on such a special day to come see me still warms my heart to this day. A year after I began treatment my uncle also fell ill with cancer but thankfully they **caught it early** and his treatment was over within a year. Our family has been through a lot over the years and I am grateful to know we were able to pull together and support each other throughout the difficult and testing times. **Also you should note:** This is why it is **so important** to support those charities that support cancer sufferers as they can be a lifeline especially to those who are not lucky enough to have such a support network as I have. **Mum, Dad, Sis, Bro #Salute!**

Family & Friends cont...

Anyone who has gone through cancer treatment or any serious illness can tell you that it is a time where you really learn who your true friends are. A lot of people fall off straight away (associates), and others fall off when the novelty wears off (fakes). I see it as a blessing because you are then left with true friends, and some people who I may not have been as close to have become my closest friends. I say fakes, you never know the reasons why people fade away they may have their own issues, but it can feel like that nevertheless.

When my body shut down I did kind of 'ghost' for a bit because I didn't want my friends seeing me in that way. What I didn't realise is some of my best healing was done whilst spending time with my friends because they made me laugh so much I just forgot about whatever I was going through at that time. My friends are so genuine and caring and they have never made me feel any different and that's why I have so much love for them.

To me it was important to maintain friendships so that I didn't lose touch with reality whilst I was living in what felt like an alternative dimension. I was often paranoid when hallucinating on the drugs so it was difficult sometimes, but they understood and have stuck by me.

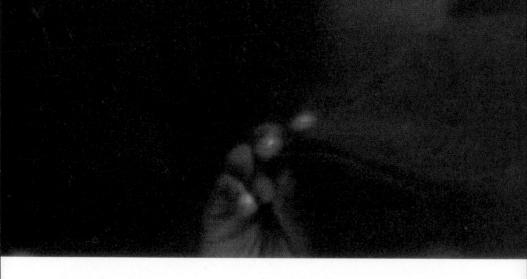

Some friendships were just not working anymore. I knew I needed to stop connecting with them. It made me feel so free and light when I did cut those ties, plus when I forgave them for how they had been it was like a negative weight had been lifted from me.

I was so nervous about meeting new people. I had always hoped they had first known the pre-cancer me. If someone watched me I would feel like they were judging me without knowing my journey. So I would find myself always telling new people my story so I could justify why I am this way. The worry is always there about how someone will react to the story. I have to say that most peoples reactions are amazing and it doesn't affect how people see me. After all these years I am finally learning that opinions don't matter and shouldn't have an effect on my life. Whatever people think and say about me is information and it's totally my choice if I absorb it or react to it.

I've made a lot of new friends who I regard as being important on my journey. Knowing that new people accepted me played a huge role in me being able to rebuild my confidence. Making new friends is just as important as maintaining current friendships. This is because essentially your character will change when you have a life changing experience and you will begin to attract like-minded people into your life.

Cancer My Summary

For me personally the cancer treatment was far worse than the actual illness. Before diagnosis I was living the life of the average teenager and besides the arm pain I looked and felt fit. Within a month after being diagnosed my mental state and physical appearance changed as a result of being on treatment.

This was scary because my whole life as I once knew it had completely changed and I felt I had lost control. Then when my whole body shut down it was even worse, but I managed to try and maintain a positive attitude. Despite this I did and can still have down days but the important thing is that I know how to pick myself back up again. Like the saying goes 'you can't have a rainbow without rain' and the bad times make you appreciate the good times even more.

Before I fell ill I would never have imagined that I would be able to cope with what I have been through. It has brought to light a whole new part of my personality; a new strength, determination and self-belief.

You can never truly know how you are going to react to a situation until it becomes your reality. Even when the doctors did not know if I'd walk again, or if I would be needing hip and or shoulder replacements... I ignored them. I chose to focus on what I believed, did my research and trusted my instincts; and in return I ended up with nothing but positive results.

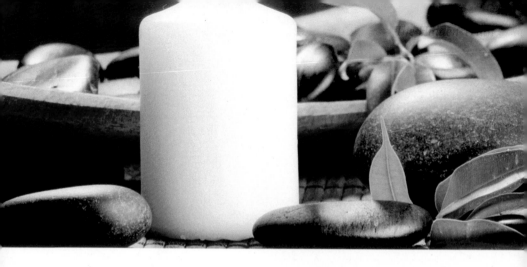

The thing is people put all their trust in to the doctors because of their qualifications and experience. This is ok to a certain extent but what people fail to remember is that no two people are the same, therefore each persons case should be treated as unique.

In my case this was especially true because the side effects were apparently so rare that none of the doctors had seen it before. So I learned that no one can know your body like you can. Only you can feel your pain and you are the one who knows when something unusual is going on with your body, so you must always try to communicate this to your medical team. Or make sure there is someone who you can rely on to speak up for you. So you tell them and they ensure your feelings are known. It is important you speak up yourself or through someone, always let them know if things are or are not improving. Everything the doctor does is based upon what you initially tell them, so if they ever tell you something can't be done just reply with "it just hasn't been done yet". If you feel there could be another way of doing something don't write your ideas off.

I faced many obstacles along the way but the trick is to never let anyone block your vision, just find the best way to get around them. The biggest thing that pushed me through my journey was... the abundance of love surrounding me and the fact that **I wanted to live and enjoy life again;** and you can!

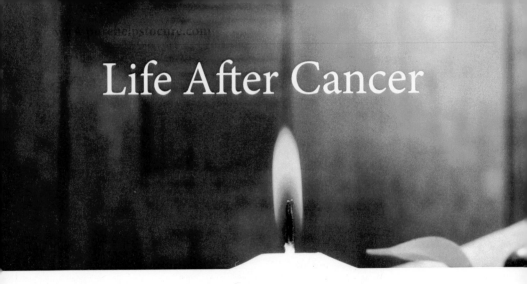

Life After Cancer

Career

For the longest time I was trying to get back to how I was before I got ill, so many factors had changed though. For years I just felt lost, not sure what I wanted to do with my life. I spent a few years doing music PR and I even set up my own digital marketing company. This was great for networking and building confidence but after a while the passion fizzled.

I kept thinking what is my purpose? I've been through cancer and some pretty horrific side effects; I've seen the patients I became close to pass away. Leaving me to ask why is it me who is still here? That's when I knew I needed to share my story in the hope that it can help and inspire others.

Maybe the things that have taken me years to work out will one day become general knowledge. My life is now based on how I can help others and make them more aware of their options. If you go through a life threatening experience it is a wake up call and has inspired me to fulfil my passions and find a purpose. Although if you are able to do this without such a painful wake up call then all the better!

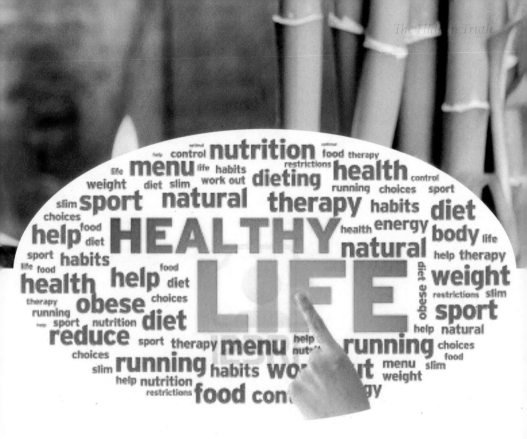

Friendships & Relationships

Even down to recently, the type of partners I am attracted to have changed. I'm attracted to the mind-set so that I know my decisions and lifestyle will be supported and understood. You shouldn't have to hide who you are because you fear others reactions. It is about being comfortable with yourself no matter what your situation is.

If people make you feel uncomfortable then you shouldn't be around each other. I distance my self from people who have a negative draining energy or don't make me feel good. I surround myself with loving, caring, positive, ambitious and like-minded people who make me laugh and feel good.

Hair & Looks

My hair grew back lovely with a softer texture and my curl pattern was a lot looser compared to before I was ill. When I had grown about an inch of hair I stopped wearing wigs and embraced my new look. I noticed that when I stopped paying attention to the length of my hair it began to grow really fast. I used to have crazy dreams about my hair being long and flowing.

My skin has been great it's really smooth and I try to only use natural products now. My skin does peel every year but it doesn't bother me because it keeps my skin feeling soft. Steroids can cause marks on the skin and I got my fair share, they have definitely decreased over the years and hopefully over time they will disappear.

The chemotherapy made my face really round and my eyes bigger. This took quite a while to go back to normal which just shows you how long these chemicals stay in your body. Gym, eating clean and detoxing the body definitely played a part in helping to get rid of the side effects.

Overall Health and Fitness

My focus has been on rehabilitation so I didn't have much time to worry about relapsing and the cancer coming back. This has really been a blessing and a welcomed distraction because I am someone who used to love to over-think things so I know I would have got quite stressed out over this.

I try to avoid taking any medication and I choose to visit my herbalist and to do holistic therapy. I have been advised by doctors to get top ups of all my jabs as the treatment wipes these from the immune system. In my eyes those jabs have way too many side effects so I would rather just strengthen my immune system by focussing heavily on my diet, lifestyle and using herbs and natural vitamins to ensure the correct nutrients are entering my body. This is a personal choice.

My whole diet has changed over the years and I try to eat only natural and organic foods as well as only really drinking water preferably warm. My rule is if there are lots of ingredients or you can't even pronounce the words in the ingredients then stay away. Once in a while I will have my cheat days but then I will try to detox myself after. I actually believe bad food is a big part of the reason why I got ill in the first place.

Exercise is a very important part of my lifestyle now and I try to do something everyday, even if it's just to go for a walk. I focus mainly on stretching the body and body weight exercises. I have been able to maintain a healthy weight and I try to focus on alignment, toning and strengthening.

My Top Tips

>>> Do things which make you happy to take your focus away from the illness

>>> Whilst you are on treatment your emotions can be up and down, don't hold them in talk to someone or write them down

>>> When you are happy and in a good mood record videos that you can watch back when you are feeling down (talk to the future you)

>>> Do lots of visualisations of yourself in a fit and healthy state

>>> Smile

>>> Keep positive

>>> Be grateful for the good things trust me you can always find some

>>> Do relaxation and meditation, just sit in silence to clear your head

>>> Listen to your heart

>>> Drink plenty of water

>>> Eat healthy pure natural and organic foods

>>> Laugh everyday

>>> Do NOT hang on to the opinions of others; remember what they say is just information and how YOU react to things determines how they will turn out not what they or anyone says

>>> Try not to react with negative emotions

>>> Remember can't just means it has not been done YET

>>> Don't let other peoples limitations become your limitations

>>> Surround yourself with positive supportive people

>>> Have a pick me up buddy(s) who you talk to when you are down

aclt

Promoting
**bone marrow &
blood donation**

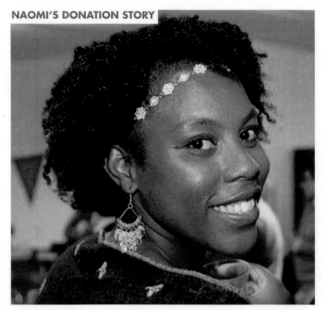

> I joined the UK stem cell register in 2005, through ACLT (African Caribbean Leukaemia Trust) whilst at Notting Hill Carnival.

I was approached by an ACLT volunteer whilst I was standing around soaking in the carnival atmosphere. They asked me if I wanted to join the stem cell register (back then it was referred to as the bone marrow register). I hadn't previously been aware such a register existed; however once I heard the volunteer speak on the woefully low numbers represented on the register for individuals of ethnic origin, it made perfect sense for me to be involved. I signed up on the spot.

Fast forward to 2007 I was contacted and informed I had come up as a match for someone. I felt so happy to know that I would be doing something so amazing. I would be saving the life of someone in need. It really was a no brainer.

In the lead up to me donating I was provided with information about the two ways in which I could donate my stem cells, the preparation involved, what happens on the day of donation and the recovery period for both options. I was then given the opportunity to decide which option I preferred to proceed with.

I decided to donate via Peripheral Blood Stem Cell donation, which is very similar to giving blood. Prior to my donation day I was given injections to stimulate the production of the blood stem cells.

In October I went ahead with the donation which mostly involved me lying down for 5 hours whilst I had my blood

NAOMI SAVING A LIFE WAS A SHORT SIMPLE PROCESS... **JUST LIKE GIVING BLOOD**

filtered. I had some minor side effects; I felt dizzy and weak however the upside was emotionally, I felt fantastic! I had completed my donation journey. Someone out there was going to receive a second chance by receiving my donation.

A few years after my donation I decided to become a volunteer for ACLT as my experience as a lifesaving donor was a wakeup call to me to support an organisation like them, in return for the support they provide to my community. Additionally my donation had me thinking about the many patients who were still in need, waiting for an unrelated stem cell matched donor to be found. I wanted to use my positive experience to encourage others to follow in my footsteps. 🙶

WE NEED MORE AFRICAN & CARIBBEAN PEOPLE TO JOIN THE STEM CELL REGISTER

When a black person with blood cancer desperately needs a lifesaving transplant they have less than a 20% chance of finding the best possible match.

YOU can improve this by joining the stem cell register. Please call ACLT on 020 3757 7700 to find out how to join the register. Or visit www.aclt.org

aclt

Promoting
bone marrow &
blood donation

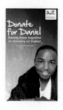 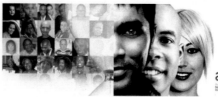

Giving Hope. Saving Lives

The ACLT (African Caribbean Leukaemia Trust) is a blood cancer charity which supports patients and their families; recruits stem cell (bone marrow), blood and organ donors; and campaigns for better services for all patients diagnosed as needing a stem cell or organ transplant.

ACLT has registered over 70,000 people of all ethnicities on to the UK stem cell registers and saved the lives of nearly 100 blood cancer patients by finding matching stem cell donors. Accumulatively, ACLT has registered nearly 100,000 potential stem cell, blood and organ donors.

The charity was co-founded in June 1996 by Beverley De-Gale OBE and Orin Lewis OBE, to find a lifesaving stem cell donor for their son, Daniel De-Gale, after he was diagnosed with acute leukaemia, and to help others fighting blood cancers and needing blood transfusions.

Why your support is needed

Someone is diagnosed with blood cancer every 20 minutes.

About 2000 people in the UK need a stem cell transplant from a stranger each year; this is usually their last chance of survival.

Bone marrow contains racially specific characteristics; the chances of finding a match are greater if the donor and patient are from the same racial background. 4 in 5 Black, mixed race and minority ethnic blood cancer patients do not find a perfect match; compared to 60%-90% for white northern European patients.

ACLT relies on the generosity of the general public to meet costs and fund activities to motivate potential lifesavers to join the stem cell, blood and organ donor registers.

How ACLT uses your donation

- To support and assist people battling leukaemia, all bone marrow related illnesses and anyone in need of an organ transplant
- To provide practical and home help, counselling, advice and moral support
- To campaign for better services for all patients diagnosed as needing a stem cell or organ transplant
- To promote stem cell, blood and organ donation

Please give from 17p a day (£5 a month) and #UniteToFightLeukaemia with ACLT

Visit www.aclt.org to make your regular or one off donation

Rest in Paradise

For all the patients I made friends with on the way but you are sadly not here today. I hope you know you are not forgotten. You understood how I felt at rock bottom. So angel in the sky who I never forget, I want you to know I am glad we met. When I think of our times together I always smile. I will see you again when it's my time to walk the final mile.

James

I met you through Naomi who is friends with my sister, and you were the first patient I spoke with. My first thought when I met you was wow this guy is full of energy and I hope I to could maintain that energy throughout my treatment. When we would talk you would never complain about anything and you didn't let your treatment get in the way of still having fun. You are truly missed and I love the way your friends and family let your legacy live on through charity fundraising days and meet ups.

Savannah

My good friend even to this day I can't believe you are gone because it came as such a shock when I found out. To my knowledge you were in remission when we last spoke and your last words to me were you telling me to keep faith and always believe. I never forgot our conversations and the jokes we would have when we were both in-patients. I miss you and your words truly inspire me to this very day. I wish I had the chance to have thanked you for bringing fun to my cancer journey. I know you see my progress... until we meet again.